And She Felt No Pain

A Japanese Doctor, His Herbal Invention, and the First General Anesthesia in Recorded History

Emily Bunker
In collaboration with Akitomo Matsuki, MD

Cover art by Nan Rae
Illustrations by Gail Brill

On the morning of October 13, she took my Mafutsusan.
A while later she became drowsy and lost consciousness.
Her whole body was numbed, and she felt no pain.

– Seishū Hanaoka
Nyūgan Chiken-roku (1805)
(*A Surgical Experience with Breast Cancer*)

A distinguished American called upon Charles Darwin, and in the
course of the conversation asked him what he considered the most
important discovery of the nineteenth century. To which Mr.
Darwin replied, after a slight hesitation: "Painless surgery."

– Frank Preston Stearns
Cambridge Sketches (1905)

"Who was first?" This is a proper pursuit because anesthesia is
one of the most valued discoveries in all of history. Few inventions
have made such a profound difference in the human condition.
The grim thought of a surgical procedure in the days when a
patient had to be awake, while a surgeon amputated a breast
or sawed through bones, is frightful to contemplate.

– Adolph H. Giesecke and Akitomo Matsuki
"Hanaoka: The Great Master of Medicine,
and His Book on Rare Diseases" (2008)

Names

Family names come before personal names in Japan. Some English language books about Japan maintain that name order, while others switch the order for westerners. This book is in the western style, as are Dr. Matsuki's books and articles that he writes in English.

Dates

Japan adopted the modern-day solar Gregorian calendar on December 3, 1872. Events before that day are dated according to the traditional Japanese calendar, which is a version of the lunisolar Chinese calendar. The difference between a date in the old calendar versus the new is about a month – sometimes less, sometimes more. (The date from the new calendar is "later.")

Macrons

Japanese in the Latin alphabet: putting a macron over a vowel (for example, "ū") is a common way to indicate that the vowel's sound is lengthened.

CONTENTS

In memory of my father, John Philip Bunker

Founding Chairman
Stanford University Department of Anesthesia

I never really knew my dad until we started writing together, the last few years of his life. One project tells the story of his 1936 high school trip to Germany, where he bicycled along the Rhine, climbed the highest mountain, saw Hitler drive by at the Olympics, and witnessed Jesse Owens win one of his four gold medals. Our other project is about his service in the U.S. Navy as a surgeon ten years later, in China and Guam.

We were always in perfect agreement – except when the topic was exclamation points. I tried a number of times to make the case that they're fine if used sparingly. Alas, my effort was in vain because he disliked them even more than the British Department for Education dislikes them. (It decided in 2016 that primary schoolchildren would get credit for using one only if the sentence began with "what" or "how.") He solemnly relented once, when I convinced him there was one spot where the punctuation mark under discussion must stay put. It was, after all, part of a title: Dad and his Navy buddies sang and danced their way through *Hopei Province!* ("a musical extravaganza based upon *Oklahoma!*") shortly before leaving China. This gem was written and accompanied on piano by fellow surgeon Abram Dansky, a graduate of Juilliard.

In the last email he sent me, a week before he died, he asked if I wanted to do something with his notes for a book that was to be about the early days of anesthesia in the West. I was thrilled, of course, and having edited some of the notes, I was already familiar with the story and his angle on it. (There's a glimpse of that angle on pages 4 and 41.) But three years later, when I got to work, I came across the *earlier* days of anesthesia in the East and was intrigued.

I didn't see any books in English for the general public about the Japanese doctor who developed and used an herbal general anesthetic, so I emailed Akitomo Matsuki, the author of the medical history book I'd just read, and suggested I write one. He welcomed the idea right away. This must have been because of who my father was, but luckily, I managed to live up to expectations. Dr. Matsuki and I worked well together.

He is the foremost scholar of Seishū Hanaoka. (He recently told me that his colleagues won't go near the subject lest they appear to be competing on "Matsuki's turf.") He sent me his latest research and his other medical history books, and then, week in and week out, let me know whenever he discovered something new.

Dad was always open to new ideas, so he would have been delighted. He ended that last email with "and we do have fun working together, don't we?" Yes, we did(!)

– E. Bunker
May 2018

Collaborator's Note

I have been studying Seishū Hanaoka since 1966, when I became a member of the Department of Anesthesiology at Hirosaki University. The shock of witnessing a fatal anesthetic accident during my internship had motivated me to go into the field, in order to study ways to prevent anesthesia-related complications. Soon after joining the department, I read W. Stanley Sykes' book *Essays on the First Hundred Years of Anaesthesia*, and was deeply impressed by the dedication. Sykes, who lost both his father and father-in-law to surgical mishaps, wrote, "In the hope that this work may help indirectly towards safer surgery. For the value of history lies in the fact that we learn by it from the mistakes of others. Learning from our own is a slow process."

Inspired by this, and by the Chinese adage "Learn wisdom from the folly of others," I was convinced that a historical approach could improve safety in the operating room. I began searching for descriptions of anesthetic injuries, eventually checking 120,000 issues of Japanese medical journals published from 1873 to 1976. It took me seventeen years because back then we didn't have computers to assist us.

I often ran across papers describing Japanese surgeon Seishū Hanaoka. Unfortunately, many of the authors – historians unfamiliar with surgery and anesthesiology – did not get the facts straight. The source of much of the information about Hanaoka is handwritten manuscripts, which can be difficult to understand. Some of them also contain errors, the result of being reproduced by hand many times over the years; it's therefore important to study the original. If it can't be found, the next best thing is to have more than one copy. Comparing multiple versions is apt to lead to a clearer understanding of what the author was trying to say.

I decided to study Hanaoka for two reasons. First, to evaluate his achievements accurately, and second, to discover how he was able to keep complications to a minimum during his thirty years of performing surgery with the general anesthetic he himself developed.

– A. Matsuki

Dr. Matsuki's note, and his abstracts in chapters 5 and 10, were edited by the author.

April 29, 2016

Dear Dr. Akitomo Matsuki,

Hello. I am the daughter of Dr. John Bunker, a well known anesthesiologist. I've just read your book *Seishū Hanaoka and His Medicine*, and would like to discuss it with you.

I am researching and writing about the early days of anesthesia. I began by reading the book my father wrote with Keith Sykes, *Anaesthesia and the Practice of Medicine: Historical Perspectives*, and then focused on the period of time when nitrous oxide, ether, and chloroform were first used as anesthetics. My research eventually took me to Seishū Hanaoka. In my opinion, a book about Dr. Hanaoka for the English-speaking general public would be an excellent idea. I think that people would be inspired by his story and medical philosophy. All of us could benefit from his example.

If you like this idea, I would be honored to be the one to take on the project. My degree is in anthropology (emphasis on linguistics and culture; my coursework included medical anthropology), which adds another dimension to my fascination with the subject. I would send you my work along the way, for your comments and corrections, and nothing would be published without your approval. Before you decide, I'd be happy to send you a sample of what I have in mind.

I look forward to hearing from you. Thank you very much.

Emily Bunker

Dear Ms. Emily Bunker,

Thank you for your mail. I am very pleased to hear that you have an interest in Seishū Hanaoka. Before starting our discussion, I should tell you that I have read the book written by Sykes and your father repeatedly and page by page. It is one of my favorite books on the history of anesthesia. The book helps me understand the western development of the specialty, and it is very important for me to balance the two ways of thinking, western and oriental.

Now I discuss the topic you raised. I welcome your proposal; it would be a great contribution to the medical profession as well as the general public. My book is only for western medical historians and not for laypeople, and it is far beyond my English ability to write for the general public. In this sense, your idea is wonderful and I think it would be welcomed. Unfortunately, many things about Hanaoka await "excavation," but only a few Japanese medical historians are studying him. To tell you the truth, I would say I am the only physician medical historian studying Hanaoka.

Before you start your project, I would like to ask you to read my chapter on Hanaoka, which appeared in my second book on the history of anesthesia in Japan. I would like to send it to you, and I shall be happy if you inform me of your postal address. My third book on the Japanese history of anesthesia is coming next February, and I can offer you the section on Hanaoka. Hoping that your project goes smoothly.

A. Matsuki, MD

For the Japanese people

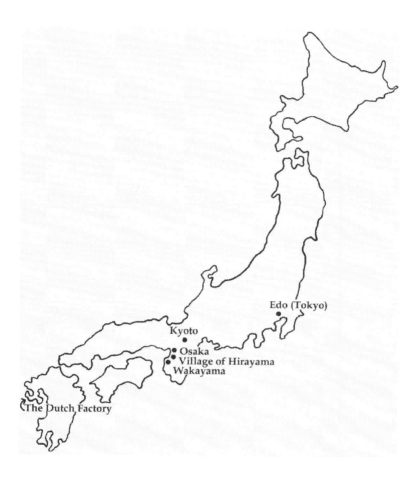

Edo (Tokyo)

Kyoto

Osaka
Village of Hirayama
Wakayama

The Dutch Factory

1. Pain Free

*When I explained my method of surgery to potential patients,
they all ran away from the hospital in fear. This woman,
however, was different. She entrusted me with her life
by allowing me to conduct the operation.*

– Seishū Hanaoka (1760-1835)

Kan Aiya swallowed a dose of *Mafutsusan* on the morning of
October 13, 1804. Within a couple of hours, she was under the
influence, ready for the tumor in her left breast to be excised.
She was willing to take a chance with the surgeon's knife and
the mysterious mixture because she was convinced it was her
last chance. Her sisters had died of the disease, and she didn't
want to be next.

Seishū Hanaoka, her doctor, was daring to try something
new. He had experimented for two decades – choosing which
herbs to include, and then tinkering with the ratios – until
magic happened. He was walking a tightrope: not far enough,
and the patient would wake up in the middle of the operation; too far, and the patient would be injured or dead.

Kan was expected to stay asleep for eight to fifteen hours.
Plenty of time. Hanaoka made an incision over the tumor and

then, using his hands, separated it from the surrounding tissues. The profuse bleeding was stopped manually. Her pulse was checked periodically. Following the removal of the tumor, the wound was cleansed, and the incision, sutured.

When she woke up, she cried, "Where is the tumor? It's gone! I'm very happy. I was never aware of the operation and felt no pain. The tumor has disappeared." She stayed at the hospital, under the care of her doctor and his assistants, until she was ready to go home a few weeks later.

Hanaoka is recognized as the first person in recorded history to perform a surgical operation with general anesthesia. Forty more years went by before anesthesia was in use in the West. To qualify as "recorded history," the record, which must be from a reliable source, has to include the surgeon's name, patient's name, date, location, and the details of the operation. This case satisfies each of these conditions. Success, of course, also depended on someone coming along who was as brave as Kan.

The news swept the country – and stopped at the borders. Japan was essentially isolated from the rest of the world, and continued to be so for another half century.

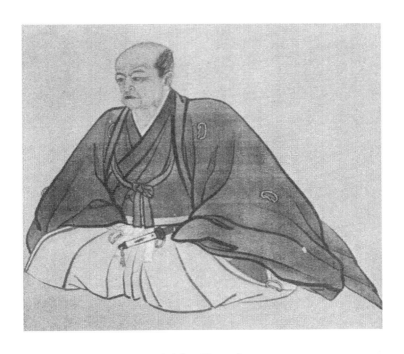

Seishū Hanaoka

2. From Boyhood

A sentence is a palanquin to carry a message of friendship.

– Seishū Hanaoka

Hanaoka wasn't concerned about his place in history. As his epitaph says:

> You were clever and brave from boyhood. You were very active in supporting people in difficult circumstances. You were honest and unaffected, and did not follow fame.

In stark contrast, battles raged in the West over who exactly had earned the title "Discoverer of Anesthesia" (the wrong question: as is often the case with discoveries and inventions, several people deserved credit). A desperate cast of characters was sidetracked by dreams of fame and fortune, and by addiction to the discoveries.

The bitter race turned a worthwhile accomplishment into a poisoned chalice, as anesthesiologist John P. Bunker put it, because what began as an untarnished gift to humanity ended up destroying most of the men who had facilitated that gift.

4

Ironically, anesthesia was already on record – though no one in the West knew – thanks to a modest Japanese man in the Land of the Rising Sun.

~

He was born on October 23, 1760, in the village of Hirayama (now Nishinoyama, Wakayama Prefecture), about three hundred miles southwest of the capital city of Edo (present-day Tokyo). On that day, his parents heard thunder and saw huge snowflakes – then it was blue skies again when their first boy was born.

Two incidents from his teen years reveal a lot about his character. At age 15, after finding a large amount of money in the road, he waited until the person it belonged to came back looking for it. When his father heard what happened, he celebrated his son's honesty with a feast for the neighbors. Another time, a troupe of actors arrived to put on a show. Seishū didn't attend because he was too busy studying, and he loved solitude. The other villagers called him an oddball who didn't know how to have fun. This didn't bother him a bit.

His medical education started with the village doctor: his father. Then, in 1782, he went to medical school. The schools with the best reputations were in Edo, Kyoto, and Nagasaki; he picked Kyoto because it was closest to home.

The Epitaph

> You had great and wise ambition, and you studied medicine diligently. As you had neither mentors nor friends with whom to discuss medicine in a secluded village like Hirayama, you went to Kyoto. You applied yourself to medicine and were absorbed in studying.

Two of his sisters, Katsu and Komutsu, earned money weaving to help make this happen. Their father was in poor health, so Seishū's sense of responsibility as the oldest son – for his seven brothers and sisters, the servants, and the neighbors whose crops were failing from recent cold weather – was one reason for his "great and wise ambition."

While in Kyoto, Seishū fell in love. He met her at a school for medicine and the koto (stringed musical instrument) that was run by his mentor Ran-en Suzuki, a famous doctor and koto player. She must have been a student of the koto because women weren't allowed to attend medical school at that time. They were both single, but when she finished school, that was the end of it. Seishū wrote her a letter and a poem:

> We were acquainted at the school of a certain scholar. A friendship sprang up between us, and strengthened day by day. It turned into love and then, at last, we moved in together. It was a joy to dine together – nothing made us happier – and whenever we took a walk, we went together. My silliness didn't make you leave

me; instead, you would gently admonish me by advising virtue with tender sentiment.

Now you're going home, and you asked me to write a Chinese poem for you. Though I'm afraid it will not be very good, how could I refuse your earnest request? A sentence is a palanquin to carry a message of friendship. If I could truly express what I want to say, I'd be a master of clarity! I ventured to compose a poem that expresses my lingering attachment to you. Please don't blame me for my poor poem. I am extremely happy.

Farewell

At the foot of a bridge, we say farewell with sorrow for parting,
As white clouds float over the faraway land where we were living.
The distant shadows of sails are swaying a thousand miles away;
All I can see is the blue sea where the edges of heaven are spreading.

3. Old-Style + Dutch-Style = Hanaoka-Style

*Recent Dutch medicine is logical in theory but rough
in practice, while Chinese medicine is fine in practice
but is wedded to ancient prescriptions.*

– Kōko Ni-ida, scholar of Chinese classics
and Seishū's friend
The Epitaph of Master Hanaoka (December 1835)

In February 1785, Hanaoka completed his education in medicine, traditional and modern, and liberal arts. The career that followed was strongly influenced by the medical philosophy of Tōdō Yoshimasu, the father of one of his teachers of traditional medicine. Yoshimasu died in 1773, but his ideas were living on through his son Nangai. They sparked Hanaoka's imagination and guided his practice for the rest of his life. He put them on his scrolls and on his licenses:

- A doctor's ultimate duty is to cure the patient.

- Mastering the art of medicine depends entirely on the individual.

- Skillfulness cannot be taught by the spoken or written word.

- We should make use of both traditional and extra-traditional formulas.

- We should study diligently our whole life.

Before he left Kyoto, his friend Keizan Asakura gave a farewell speech that included these words:

> Seishū Hanaoka tirelessly read not only medical and surgical texts but also the Chinese classics of ethics, politics, and Taoism. He understood their significance. He sought the advice of famous doctors who had profound knowledge and skills.

Hanaoka had hoped to learn the latest innovations in Kyoto, but he concluded that "old-style" (traditional Chinese) medicine should be more progressive, and "Dutch-style" (modern western) medicine was not living up to its promises. Meanwhile, as each side vied for public acceptance, scholar Gentaku Ōtsuki was insisting that the "two systems of medicine could be complementary, each overcoming the inadequacies of the other." Later, in a March 28, 1815, letter to Hanaoka, Ōtsuki told him he was "the number one surgeon in Asia" and that he had "exquisite technique and divine skill."

That letter made him realize he had established a unique style of surgery: "Hanaoka-style."

His success was due in part to having correctly assessed the medical world when the time came to find his place in it. East and West were converging in Japan, and he envisioned the seemingly opposite styles coexisting in harmony:

> If you want to practice modern surgery, you should learn traditional medicine first. Otherwise, your results will not be good. Let's say someone has a carbuncle; the correct remedy should lead to a rapid recovery. But the carbuncle won't be cured even days later if you only treat it surgically, and sometimes the patient will die.

And as described by the author of his epitaph:

> Medicine is now divided into traditional and Dutch, and under these circumstances a patient is not cured. You, on the other hand, insisted, "When we treat our patients, we should combine herbs according to their symptoms; it is not always necessary to follow traditional prescriptions. When herbs are not effective, acupuncture can be applied. If acupuncture doesn't bring the expected results, we should perform surgery."

Why "Dutch" medicine? A multilayered link between Japan and the Netherlands developed during the two centuries that twenty or so Dutch men were stationed on (and restricted to) a 2.2-acre manmade island in Nagasaki Harbor. The island had been carved from the end of a peninsula into the shape of a fan, then reconnected to the mainland by a heavily guarded bridge. It was the avenue for western medicine. The only avenue. But before *that* surprising story is told . . .

A thousand years earlier, a blind Chinese Buddhist priest named Jian Zhen tried five times in twelve years to cross the choppy East China Sea in order to spread Buddhism in Japan. He finally made it in 754. An expert in herbal medicine, he brought herbs along with him and taught the Japanese priests how to use them. And because of his excellent sense of smell, his blindness didn't keep him from being able to tell one from the other. Chinese medicine had already been introduced to Japan via Korea, but now, because of Jian Zhen's dedication and free healthcare services, it was firmly established. *Ishinhō* (*The Essence of Medicine and Therapeutic Methods*), a compilation of Chinese medical knowledge, was published in Japan in 984.

Over time, old-style medicine was adapted to Japanese culture, independent of China, with two completely different philosophies. The Kohōha School (School of Classical Formulas) was the method Hanaoka studied. It advocated choosing a remedy based on the symptoms – that is, focusing on what can be observed – without mixing in unproven theories about the human body. Tōyō Yamawaki, of the Kohōha School, was the first doctor in Japan to perform a human dissection with official permission. The dissection took place in 1754, and in 1759, the year before Hanaoka was born, Yamawaki's illustrated book *Zōshi* (*Explanations of Internal Organs*) came out. It revealed that the proponents of the theoretical approach were wrong about the appearance of the inside of the body.

Twelve years later, doctors Genpaku Sugita and Ryōtaku Ma-eno, unsatisfied with the primitive illustrations in *Zōshi*, thought they should see for themselves. They got permission to witness the dissection of a decapitated criminal at the execution site in Edo (Tokyo) on March 4, 1771.

Coincidentally, each had with him a copy of *Ontleedkundige Tafelen* (*Anatomical Tables*), the 1734 Dutch translation of an anatomy book by German medical lecturer Johann Adam Kulmus. As the men had suspected – although it was still astonishing to observe firsthand – the organs in the corpse's thorax and abdomen matched the illustrations in the Dutch book, rather than the illustrations they were familiar with in Chinese anatomy textbooks. (The errors were rooted in Confucianism: in ancient China the body was sacred, so surgery and dissection were thought to be forms of mutilation.)

Ontleedkundige Tafelen, they decided, must be translated. Knowing some Dutch already, they (with two others) did it themselves; since Ma-eno was the most proficient, he was in charge. After three challenging years without the luxury of a

Dutch-Japanese dictionary, inventing Japanese vocabulary for various parts of the anatomy along the way, Sugita, Ma-eno, et al. published the five-volume *Kaitai Shinsho* (*New Text on Anatomy*) in 1774. This book went on to have an enormous influence on the acceptance of western medicine in Japan.

All of which, as mentioned, entered through that tiny fan-shaped island off the coast of Nagasaki.

Its name was Dejima ("exit island"); colloquially, it was known as the Dutch Factory. The island was a Dutch trading post from 1641 until Japan's self-imposed isolation ended, a little over two hundred years later. In the beginning, it was run by Vereenigde Oost-Indische Compagnie (United East India Company). Then, when the company went bankrupt in 1796, by the Dutch government. For a few years in the early nineteenth century, during the Napoleonic Wars, it was the only place on Earth flying the Dutch flag.

The Dutch presence began on April 19, 1600, when one of their ships washed ashore. The twenty-four starving sailors had been at sea for two years, on a mission to raid and plunder Spanish and Portuguese settlements across the globe for pepper, a prized commodity, and other spices. All the sailors were Dutch except for the English captain, Will Adams. (A fictionalized version of Adams is the hero of the 1975 novel *Shōgun* by James Clavell.)

The Portuguese were already there. They arrived in 1543, and were welcomed because of what they were selling: firearms. But when their interest in political and religious power became clear, the warm welcome evaporated. Christian missionaries were expelled in 1614. By 1639, all westerners except the Dutch had left, voluntarily or otherwise.

Japan was closing its doors, which the government decided was necessary for the sake of national security. From 1792 to 1849, Russia, England, and the United States all tried and failed to secure even the right to provisions for their ships at Japanese ports. Then, in July 1853, U.S. Commodore Matthew C. Perry arrived with orders from Millard Fillmore, the previous U.S. President, to force Japan open – for trade, for provisions and fuel, and for better treatment of castaways. (The Netherlands suspected this was going to happen, and alerted Japan in 1852, but the warning was ignored.) The Treaty of Kanagawa was signed on March 31, 1854, and the country was closed no longer. Hanaoka rose to fame in the last fifty years of the period of isolation.

~

From the start, the Dutch merchants were perceived as trustworthy, with no interest in meddling in politics or religion. It also helped that they didn't get along with the Portuguese. As foreigners, however, they still must be monitored. (Before the isolation policy went into effect, they essentially had free rein, as did the other westerners.) The island was built for the Portuguese, to keep them under the government's watchful eye – but they'd barely settled in when they were sent away. What about their nice new home? The Dutch got it.

According to legend, the fan idea came from the Shōgun; when asked what the future trading post should look like, he supposedly whipped out his fan and said, "Like this!"

Thus began the way out for Japanese silver, gold, copper, camphor, lacquerware, porcelain, and tea, and the way in for Chinese silk, among many other things. Coffee and chocolate. Beer, badminton, and billiards. The very first camera arrived aboard a Dutch ship in 1848. (The abrupt reversal of Japan's relationship to the outside world a couple of years later made it pointless to funnel imports and exports through a narrow passageway – so cameras started pouring into the country.) The islanders could also do a little of their own trading on the side: a convenient way to earn some extra money.

Japanese citizens, other than a handful of officials, translators, and doctors, were not allowed into the Dutch Factory. And the factory workers weren't allowed out, except for the periodic visit to Edo to demonstrate their loyalty, offer gifts such as telescopes, globes, medical instruments, and the occasional camel/monkey/zebra – they were given expensive silk kimonos in return – and to bring news from abroad. Reporting the events of the day is considered to have been Dejima's primary function. Moreover, by isolating the messengers, the government believed it had strict control of the information. That idea was doomed. People find a way to talk.

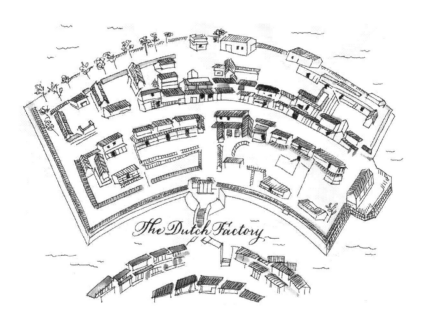

The Dutch Factory

Since Japanese artists hardly, if ever, caught sight of the exotic foreigners, they resorted to guesswork. They settled on painting them – practically all of them! – with red hair, blue eyes, and big noses.

Caspar Schamberger, of Germany, was the first European doctor to serve there. He arrived in 1649 and stayed two and a half years, inspiring the first western medical school in Japan in the process. "Caspar-style" (or rather, *Kasuparu*-style) surgery had a powerful effect on Hanaoka's own style.

Two doctor-scientists stationed on Dejima who contributed greatly to the exchange of knowledge between Japan and the western world were Engelbert Kaempfer (on the island from 1690 to 1692) and Philipp Franz von Siebold (from 1823 to 1829). Both were German. Kaempfer, who quickly became fluent in Japanese and made many friends as a result, was a naturalist who would have preferred to be free to explore the countryside on his own (although doctors had more freedom than the other "red-haired barbarians"). He helped introduce soybeans to the West. Siebold is noted for his writings about Japanese flora and fauna, and for his book *Nippon* (seven volumes, published from 1832 to 1882), a comprehensive description of nineteenth century Japan.

Siebold's stay ended dramatically when he was arrested and deported for trying to smuggle secret maps and other forbidden items out of the country. (He returned thirty years later.) The scandal, which had deadly and far-reaching consequences, came to be known as the Siebold Incident.

Books in Dutch covering a wide range of subjects crossed over the bridge. The ability to read and translate the language became a valuable skill due to its sudden status as the *lingua franca* with the West, and because it was a stepping stone to other languages that use the Latin alphabet. This jerry-rigged information highway served the medical world more than any other: circumventing language barriers and national borders is worth the trouble when the result is knowledge that can save or improve lives.

The Epitaph

> You integrated several theories. You used traditional methods but were not trapped. You created new methods but did not forget tradition. You could cure even rare and intractable diseases that are not described in textbooks.

There had been earlier attempts in Japan to integrate the old and the new, but Hanaoka-style medicine achieved the perfect balance. At times, the approach confused people, and he didn't like that:

> I am an expert in traditional medicine, but people say I specialize in modern surgery. I am unhappy with these inadequate words!

4. Fish Hooks or Finger Traps

My medical skill is a spontaneous response of my hands to what comes into my head, so it's difficult to express this process in words.

– Seishū Hanaoka

A boy from a faraway village with a fish hook stuck deep in his throat was taken, in desperation, to the renowned Seishū Hanaoka. Others had tried to remove the hook by pulling on the line hanging from his mouth. Hanaoka quickly sized up the situation, then asked one of his students to find and break an abacus. He threaded the abacus beads onto the fishing line until they lay in a row to form a stick. No laryngoscope was available back then, so, working blind, he gently guided the stick of beads down the lucky little boy's throat until the hook came loose.

This predicament brings to mind a toy called the Chinese finger trap: a woven bamboo cylinder used for practical jokes. They're about 5 inches long, with the circumference of a human finger. If you are the innocent victim, you have been instructed to put a finger into each end of the cylinder, and then to take your fingers out. Easy, right? Not if you're like most people. Chances are, you will simply pull – to no avail. But if you push your fingers *farther in*, the trap will widen, relaxing its grip and setting you free.

~

The scalpel's cutting and scraping was merely excruciating. The red-hot iron used for cauterizing (as yet, the best way to stop bleeding) hurt even more. Those who were critically ill or injured braced themselves for emergency surgery, thinking they would die otherwise.

Elective surgery candidates, on the other hand, weren't so sure. Hanaoka was hoping for a day when surgeon and prospective patient could thoroughly discuss the options; then, if surgery was requested, the operation could proceed at a comfortable pace. Impossible if said patient is feeling each twist of the knife. Operating at full tilt – to reduce the time spent being traumatized – would be a thing of the past. His goal was to simultaneously erase pain and awareness (today's definition of general anesthesia), not only so there'd be no pain, but no memory of the experience either.

A variety of herbal formulas for abdominal and muscular pain was already available. And getting drunk before surgery was not unheard of. But none of this was powerful enough to give dependable relief. Anesthesiologists Adolph H. Giesecke and Akitomo Matsuki discuss perspectives on surgical pain in their article "Hanaoka: The Great Master of Medicine, and His Book on Rare Diseases":

> Hanaoka was unique in his attitude toward the suffering of his patients, especially those requiring surgery. Surgeons of the time in the West believed that the pain of surgery counteracted shock and improved recovery. The pain of surgery was part of the process, and one had to "take it like a man." By contrast, Hanaoka felt that it was his duty to spare the patients from the pain that other doctors could not relieve. He believed that good sedation was indispensable to reduce suffering, facilitate the operation and minimize danger to the patient.

The following passage – from Dokushōan Nagatomi's 1764 book *Man-yū Zakki* (*Miscellaneous Travel Notes*) – was a factor in his decision to focus on breast cancer:

> Breast cancer has been incurable since olden times. In a western medical textbook, they say the cancer can be excised when the tumor is the size of an apricot seed and in the initial stage of development. As I have not yet tried this excision, I mention it here, with the hope that future trials will be performed by younger generations.

Knowing that western surgeons were operating without anesthesia, Hanaoka scoffed at such an idea . . .

It is said that Dutch surgeons pinch a breast cancer tumor with a pair of large shears, such as those used by blacksmiths. Patients would be dead after an operation like that. This story is a lie.

. . . and was spurred on to his eventual breakthrough:

Although breast cancer is considered incurable, I always believed that a hundred patients out of a hundred would not necessarily succumb to the disease, and that an effective treatment could allow one or two patients out of ten to avoid death.

~

The fish hook story demonstrates that Hanaoka not only had a knack for applying familiar principles in new ways, but also an understanding that we cannot always depend on our instincts to tell us how to "go forward." A willingness to try the illogical route enables escapes from fish hooks and finger traps – and it enabled an escape, at that time in history, from the agony of surgery without anesthesia. Hanaoka incorporated elements of traditional Chinese medicine into modern western surgical techniques, causing a paradigm shift on the operating room table. In short, he could go forward because first, he went back.

No longer would patients undergoing surgery need to be held in place by a team of strong men, or relegated to distant corners of the hospital so that nobody would have to listen to the bloodcurdling screams.

~

Studying, modifying, and finding inspiration in ancient herbal formulas was the route he took to put an end to the misery in modern-day surgery. At first glance, the escape plan might seem a trifle counterintuitive, if not downright unbelievable. Unless you're familiar with fish hooks or finger traps.

5. Traces of an Invention

A simultaneous use of scopolamine (Datura) and aconitine (Aconitum) offsets the side effects of both and provides a synergetic effect of analgesia and loss of consciousness. This is the very result that Seishū must have taken great pains to discover.

– Akitomo Matsuki
Seishū Hanaoka and His Medicine:
A Japanese Pioneer of Anesthesia and Surgery

Traces left by those who preceded Hanaoka provide clues to the origins and development of his herbal invention. The predecessors' insights, knowledge, and experiments laid the foundation for Hanaoka to put together the rest of the puzzle. One such trace was left by his contemporary Nan-yō Hara, whose detailed pharmacological description of *Datura* in his collection of clinical experiences, *Sōkei Gūki* (1798), was a significant contribution to the process. Here are a few lines of a Chinese poem Hanaoka wrote for Hara (whom he never did meet), expressing his gratitude:

Living under the sky a thousand miles apart, I know you by name only. Your book came by way of the sea; it conveys new knowledge, expanding my ideas. Some day in the near future I will invite you to my grove to enjoy a conversation, while we drink to springtime.

Uncovering the full story of these traces isn't easy because Hanaoka left behind few notes, and he didn't publish. Separating fact from hearsay, to which Matsuki has been dedicated since 1966, is therefore painstaking work. This research includes traveling around the country to view manuscripts and scrolls in archives and libraries. He writes passages down by hand because photocopies and photographs are generally not allowed.

Other traces were left by anesthesia pioneers Senzō Hanai and Harunobu Ōnishi of Kyoto. Their formulas were similar to *Mafutsusan* – in particular, all three contained the same two key herbs – so their work clearly contributed to it. Hanaoka might have met Ōnishi, but evidently not Hanai because he is thought to have died by the end of 1781, the year before Hanaoka moved to Kyoto for medical school.

The path taken by Hanai and Ōnishi began with an herbal formula, *Sō-u-san*, that was described in a 1337 Chinese medical book called *Shiyi Dexiao Fang* in Chinese and *Sei-i-tokko-ho* in Japanese, and in *A Bone Setting Handbook* (1746) by Hōyoku Takashi. The primary purpose of *Sō-u-san* was pain relief for broken bones and dislocated joints. Its recipe was complex, with fourteen herbs, so one of the changes Hanai made was reducing the number of ingredients. Ōnishi's prescription is a modification of Hanai's.

According to *A List of Anesthetic Formulas Related to Seishū Hanaoka* (1971) by Hajime Sōda, Hanaoka started by refining Hanai's prototype. He later explored the findings of anesthesia investigators Sadakichi Iwanaga, Kinkei Nakagami, and Genkitsu Yoshio. More traces. Any of these men might have used something that approximated general anesthesia, and, even if they missed the mark, pain and awareness might have been at least partially eliminated. None of them documented anything, however, probably due to the traditional secrecy in medicine (more on this topic in chapter 11).

The art of observation and experimentation, which Hanaoka had learned from his training in traditional Chinese medicine, no doubt contributed to his willingness to go slowly. Some of this time was spent bringing the number of herbs down to six, for simplicity's sake; he added two and removed four from Hanai's formula. There was also the monumental task of determining the best ratios. By trial and error – using himself and other intrepid volunteers – he searched for that elusive boundary between safety on the one hand and effectiveness on the other. Complicating things further, in practice he'd have to be able to adjust the ratios on the spot, as needed by the individual patient.

But since he was a cautious scientist, he was in no great hurry to put *Mafutsusan* to the test in the operating room. If he'd cared about being The First, rather than simply helping people who were sick or injured, chances are he would have gone ahead with surgery under general anesthesia a lot earlier than 1804. After all, by 1796 he was very close. The following is from Matsuki's abstract about his research on the manuscript *Mayaku Kō* (*A Treatise on Anesthetics*), which describes the evolution of the search for anesthesia in Japan:

> Seishū Hanaoka's greatest achievement was the oral general anesthetic *Mafutsusan*. He developed it, and then used it successfully for various operations, primarily breast cancer tumor excisions. The developmental process is described in *Mayaku Kō*, a manuscript written and edited in 1796 by Hanaoka's close friend Shūtei Nakagawa. Contained in the document is a list of fourteen prescriptions for earlier attempts by other doctors to create general and topical anesthetics. These prescriptions, which Nakagawa had passed along to Hanaoka, were the foundation for the scientific breakthrough. The preface suggests that he had nearly perfected *Mafutsusan* by 1796.

The original *Mayaku Kō* is gone (it wasn't published; however, a plagiarized version called *Hiyaku Kō* was published in 1826), but seven handwritten copies have been located, five of them by Matsuki. He has been studying the manuscript since 1983, when he found his first copy.

The idea for the project came about in 1788, when Nakagawa's house in Kyoto burned down. Hanaoka invited his friend to stay with him until he got back on his feet; during that time they discussed the medical issues of the day, including the hot topic of the hunt for anesthesia.

Their discussions segued to Nakagawa searching medical books for prescriptions for previous attempts, then putting it all together in *Mayaku Kō* in May 1796. Although *Mafutsusan* was indeed producing the desired effect by that time, the inventor didn't think his invention was ready to accompany an operation. It probably caused a light state of unconsciousness, without an ironclad guarantee to erase pain. Throughout the years of refining his anesthetic, Hanaoka did practice surgery, but minor procedures only because he didn't want to subject anyone to something major without sedation.

From Nakagawa's Preface to Mayaku Kō

In our country, Hanai was a pioneer. He created several prescriptions, and experimented for a long time, but it has been said that in the end he didn't develop an effective anesthetic. In recent years, many doctors have been concerned with anesthetics, and carefully scrutinized them. Sadakichi Iwanaga [one of Hanaoka's teachers] of Kyoto had some good ideas. A student of his implored him to reveal his prescription, but he would not. The student then tried to develop his own formula, but none was effective. Hakkō Hanaoka [one of Seishū's names; it was used by his friends], a friend of mine, has had a longstanding involvement with surgery, and has unceasingly studied how to alleviate surgical pain. He finally developed an effective preparation. I observed him administer his general anesthetic to more than ten volunteers, and it worked for all of them.

I have described here the prescriptions for anesthetics, which I've collected for widespread use. I hope readers will investigate them.

The *Mayaku Kō* formulas were placed in one of three categories, depending on whether they contained *Datura*, *Aconitum*, or both. Iwanaga used *Datura* but not *Aconitum*. He tested his formula with breast cancer surgery, but his patients died soon after, so he gave up.

Hanaoka came to realize that *Datura* without *Aconitum* would not provide a sufficient amount of pain relief, and that the dose required to induce general anesthesia could be deadly. The presence of *Aconitum* made such a big dose unnecessary (although *Mafutsusan* still contained much more *Datura* than anything else). He also investigated *Aconitum* without *Datura*, but rejected that idea as potentially deadly as well.

Datura and *Aconitum* are the key herbs referenced in the beginning of this chapter. Hanaoka discovered that it wasn't simply a matter of what each contributed: when put together, the plants work synergistically in both their effectiveness and their safety. In other words, in the *Mafutsusan* formula, these two ingredients were greater than the sum of their parts.

Finding the ideal ratio was wildly difficult. Neither Hanai nor Ōnishi could figure it out, and it was still eluding Hanaoka in 1796. *Datura* played a smaller role at that time than it ultimately did; in the final version, the ratio of *Datura* to *Aconitum* fluctuated between 3:1 and 4:1, depending on the patient's needs.

- *Datura* enhanced the analgesic effect of *Aconitum*, and *Aconitum* enhanced the sedative effect of *Datura*.

- *Datura*, which causes tachycardia (fast heartrate), counteracted the bradycardia (slow heartrate) that *Aconitum* causes – and vice versa.

- The four other herbs rounded out the effect.

6. Six Potent Plants

Hanaoka's anesthesia was an over-dosage of several alkaloids, including scopolamine, atropine, aconitine and angelicotoxin. When combined, these ingredients induce hypnosis, analgesia, muscle weakness and lack of recall. We would compare it to "very heavy sedation."

– Adolph H. Giesecke and Akitomo Matsuki

Alkaloids are medicinally active chemicals made primarily by plants. Examples are caffeine, strychnine, ephedrine, quinine, codeine, nicotine, and cocaine. They've been in use since ancient times, and many have anesthetic properties. Scopolamine is the most powerful alkaloid in *Datura*; general anesthesia by means of *Mafutsusan* is chiefly the result of its effect on the central nervous system. Aconitine is the most powerful alkaloid in *Aconitum*.

Detailed plant information can be found at Plants For A Future, a charitable organization in Cornwall, England. With a database of over seven thousand species, it researches and provides information on plants, "particularly those which have edible, medicinal or other uses." This is what they say about *Mafutsusan*'s six potent plants:

Datura alba Nees

Usual *Mafutsusan* ratio part: 6-8
Logo of the Japanese Society of Anesthesiologists

Synonyms: *Datura alba* and *Datura metel L*
Common names: Thorn Apple, Angel's Trumpet,
Hindu *Datura*, Horn of Plenty, Downy Thorn Apple
An annual that grows to 1.5 meters
Native to southern China and India;
naturalized in the Mediterranean

A poultice of the crushed leaves of *Datura alba Nees* is used for pain relief. The whole plant (but leaves and seed especially) is anesthetic, anodyne (relieves pain), anti-asthmatic, antispasmodic, antitussive (prevents coughing), hypnotic, hallucinogenic, mydriatic (causes pupil dilation), and a bronchodilator. Used to treat asthma in China, and to treat epilepsy, hysteria, insanity, heart disease, fever with catarrh (excessive mucus), diarrhea, and skin diseases in India. The flowers and leaves are dried and used in anti-asthmatic cigarettes in Vietnam.

While the flowers have an exotic fragrance, the bruised leaves have an unpleasant smell.

Great caution is advised since it can cause hallucinations, severe intoxication, and death. The medicinal dose is perilously close to the toxic dose, so this plant should only be used under the supervision of a qualified practitioner.

All members of this genus contain narcotics and are very poisonous, even in small doses.

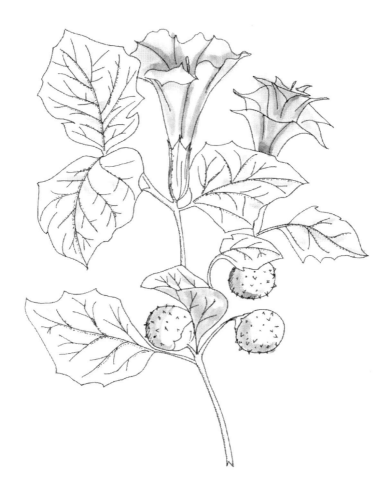

Datura alba Nees

Aconitum japonicum
Usual *Mafutsusan* ratio part: 2

A perennial that grows to 1 meter by .3 meter
Native to Japan and China

The root of *Aconitum japonicum,* a widely used Chinese herbal remedy, is analgesic, stimulant, anti-rheumatic, and cardio-tonic (stimulates the heart). Used in the treatment of neural-gia (facial nerve pain).

Inhibits the growth of nearby species, especially legumes, and thrives in most soils. Members of this genus seem to be im-mune to the predations of rabbits and deer.

The whole plant is highly toxic; simple skin contact can cause numbness. It should only be used under the supervision of a qualified practitioner.

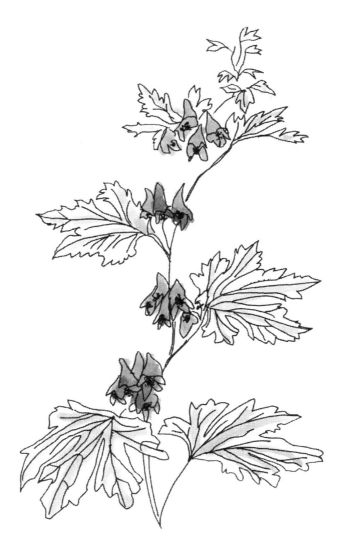

Aconitum japonicum

Angelica dahurica

Usual *Mafutsusan* ratio part: 1

Common name: Bai Zhi
A biennial/perennial that grows to 1.8 meters
Native to Japan, Korea, and Siberia

Angelica dahurica has been used for thousands of years in Chinese herbal medicine as a sweat-inducing herb to counter harmful external influences. Used to treat frontal headaches, toothaches, rhinitis, boils, carbuncles, and skin diseases. Induces vomiting, decreases pulse, and increases blood pressure, rate of respiration, and secretion of saliva. Contraindicated for pregnant women.

All members of this genus contain furocoumarins (chemical compounds produced by a variety of plants), which increase skin sensitivity to sunlight and may cause dermatitis. In large doses can cause convulsions and generalized paralysis.

Angelica acutiloba

Usual *Mafutsusan* ratio part: 1

Common name: Dong Dang Gui
A perennial that grows to .7 meter
Native to Japan and China; in particular,
the mountains of central Japan

The root of *Angelica acutiloba* is an emmenagogue (stimulates menstrual flow), oxytocic (stimulates childbirth contractions), sedative, and tonic. Eases dizziness.

May cause dermatitis for the same reason as *Angelica dahurica*.

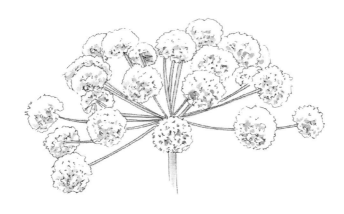

Angelica dahurica

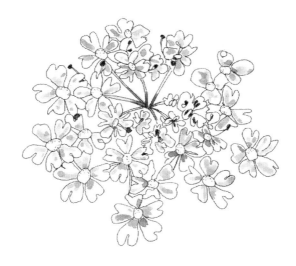

Angelica acutiloba

Arisaema japonicum

Usual *Mafutsusan* ratio part: 2

Synonym: *Arisaema serratum*
A perennial that grows to .9 meter
Native to Japan, China, and Korea;
in particular, shady forests in central and southern Japan

The root of *Arisaema japonicum* is alterative (restores health), de-obstruent (removes obstructions), discutient (dissipates diseased matter), vulnerary (heals wounds), diuretic, and an expectorant.

Contains calcium oxalate crystals, which can feel like needles sticking into the mouth and tongue if the plant is eaten. Easily neutralized, however, by thoroughly drying or cooking the plant, or by steeping it in water. Use with caution.

Cnidium officinale

Usual *Mafutsusan* ratio part: 2

A perennial that grows to .5 meter
Native to China

The root of *Cnidium officinale* is analgesic, antibacterial, anti-convulsive, anti-inflammatory, hypotensive, sedative, a vaso-dilator, and a febrifuge (reduces fever). Used mainly to treat headaches; also dysmenorrhea (painful menstruation), amen-orrhea (absence of menstruation), cerebral embolism, coro-nary heart disease, pain, and weakness.

At least one member of this genus has a report of toxicity so caution is advised.

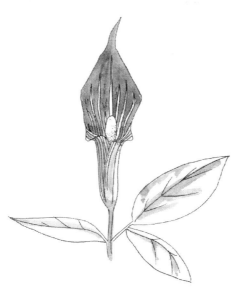

Arisaema japonicum

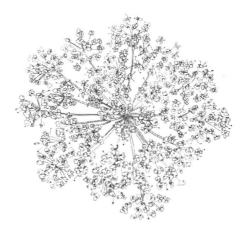

Cnidium officinale

7. Testing, Testing

Both of my legs were paralyzed . . .

– Seishū Hanaoka

Hanaoka experimented with his creation on himself, and on the family members, friends, and students who volunteered as test subjects. No surgery; they were just seeing how well it worked. The men took their dose of the powdered anesthetic-in-progress dissolved in sake (fermented liquor). The women took it with water. It might have been tested on animals too, but no documentation exists to verify this.

His wife, Ka-e Imose (1762-1829), with whom he had six children, was rumored to have volunteered for the experiments, possibly going blind from long-term exposure to the powerful herbs. His mother, Otsugi, might also have participated. *The Doctor's Wife* is the name of the English translation of a popular 1966 book by Sawako Ariyoshi. It was made into a movie in 1967. This fictional story about Ka-e, Otsugi, and the *Mafutsusan* experiments was the sole source of Hanaoka information for the majority of the Japanese people. It therefore was, and still is, widely believed to be a true story.

Self-experimentation is a longstanding scientific tradition. That was the approach taken by some anesthesia pioneers in the West in the 1840s, before they understood how addictive those drugs are. A few lost their minds and then their lives. One of them took his own life, in prison, because he couldn't live with what he had done while under the influence of chloroform.

Hanaoka evidently paid a price as well: his legs were paralyzed from September to September 1803-04. His repeated experiments on himself may or may not have been the cause of the paralysis, but either way, the result was a delay in testing *Mafutsusan* with surgery. He wrote the following on New Year's Day 1805:

> From autumn 1803 to autumn 1804 I lay on my sickbed. Both of my legs were paralyzed, and it was difficult to walk without a cane. When the poison that caused the paralysis was exhausted, I completely recovered from my illness. I composed two Chinese poems, four lines each and seven characters per line, to celebrate my recovery and this tranquil village.

Mafutsusan was ready by the end of 1803; about nine months later its inventor was ready too. Three women had made appointments at Shunrinken – Hanaoka's hospital and medical school, situated in his village, Hirayama – between January and June 1804, in order to find out what breast cancer surgery entailed. All three got scared and ran home.

Then Kan showed up.

8. Kan Gets Her Wish

Doctor, you know how to treat this disease, so please do not hesitate to make me the subject of your surgery. If I visit the land of the dead because of it, I will never cry over it.

– Kan Aiya (1745-1805)

Kan's trailblazing story was well documented, so it left much more than a trace. Since the summer of '03, she'd been aware of a lump in her left breast. She consulted multiple doctors, and they all diagnosed breast cancer too far along for any treatment they were capable of providing. Time passed, and the tumor got bigger. She was advised to make an appointment with a certain famous doctor . . .

From Hanaoka's Case Report

A woman named Kan Aiya came to me complaining, "Last summer, I became aware of a swelling in my left breast. I could feel a lump the size of a bean, which gradually grew to the size of a *Go* stone [the playing pieces used in the ancient game of *Go*; they're about 22 millimeters in diameter]. I consulted with several doctors; they all diagnosed the lump as breast cancer, and refused to provide treatment because they thought it was incurable. I lived without hope for a year and a half. Meanwhile, the lump kept growing bigger. Then someone asked, 'Haven't you heard the name Seishū Hanaoka, who can take care of rare diseases? Why are you letting time slip away, only to accept death? You should go visit him and request treatment.' So I came here in a hurry to consult with you. I hope you will do me this favor. Nothing would make me happier than to survive by your treatment, which offers the chance of one life in ten deaths."

I examined her. I saw that her left breast was swollen, and her skin was tinged darkish at 5 centimeters from the nipple, under which a tumor was palpable. It was the size of a teacup and as hard as a *Go* stone. She complained of neither pain nor itching, but there was stiffness in her left shoulder, and pain sometimes radiated to her chest.

This was indeed breast cancer. *Waikezhengzong* [a Chinese textbook published in 1617] describes it as follows: melancholy suppresses the function of the liver, and prudence impedes that of the spleen. When a great deal of discontent accumulates in a woman's heart and is not resolved, the spirits become congested and form a tumor in her breast. The tumor is initially the size of a *Go* stone. In half a year, then in one, two, and three years, it grows bigger without aching. It is later accompanied by continuous pain. Day by day, it becomes the size of a Japanese chestnut, and then a teacup. The skin over the tumor is darkish, and an ulcer develops that is deeply pitted at first, and then convex; at that stage it looks like a wilting lotus flower. Pain radiates to the chest, and the blood from the tumor is malodorous. Eventually, the five viscera deteriorate, and the patient cannot be cured. [The five viscera are the heart, lungs, liver, spleen, and kidneys. The phrase generally means the entire body.]

Waikebaixiao Quanshu [another Chinese textbook; publication date unknown] says this: if anger accumulates, liver and spleen dysfunctions will result, causing a tumor the size of a *Go* stone to form in the breast. At first, there is no pain or itching. In five to seven years, the skin over the tumor turns black-purple, and an ulcer gradually develops inside the tumor. Breast cancer incurs death by exhausting all energy and blood.

"Do your best and leave the rest to Providence" is an old proverb. Who could blame me for not resuscitating someone if the treatment might cause death, even if one or two patients out of ten could have recovered? I was anxious because there was no experience with breast cancer surgery in our country or in China. Many years ago I saw an illustration of a surgical operation of the breast in a western textbook, and have been thinking about the method ever since. Finally, I had a divine revelation. It's hard to treat a patient when the tumor is already ulcerated, and the skin over the tumor is already black-purple. The tumor in Kan's left breast, however, was not yet ulcerated, and her skin was not black-purple, indicating she could be treated surgically.

On the other hand, since it is widely believed that diseases considered incurable should not be treated rashly, I told her I wasn't ready yet.

She replied, "Doctor, please do not refuse me. I know that breast cancer is very difficult to cure; I've been aware of that from the beginning. My sisters suffered from the disease, but doctors rejected them, and ulcerated tumors led to their deaths. I closely observed this. Now I am suffering from the same disease, and I know the treatment is not easy. Not treating it might lead to a longer life but would prolong the agony. Treating it might invite death, but the agony would end. It would be better for me to urge death to escape the torment than to live longer in anguish. I discussed my decision with my family, and then came here. Doctor, you know how to treat this disease, so please do not hesitate to make me the subject of your surgery. If I visit the land of the dead because of it, I will never cry over it."

This woman was quite prepared for surgery. I said, "Although I won't carry out the operation at present, I will try it someday. I do not obstinately refuse to do it." I explained to her, "My method of treating breast cancer follows that of Huà Tuó [see chapter 9]. Exposing the tumor will bring loss of consciousness upon you. Every condition you have should therefore be alleviated, and your spirit and energy should be well balanced. After that, I will perform the surgery. You're suffering from the pain of beriberi [thiamine deficiency]. This must be treated first." I wrote a prescription for *Keisikajutsubutō* [an herbal remedy] and said to her, "Take this, and you will recover from your beriberi. Be sure to see me again, and I will take care of your breast cancer as soon as possible."

The patient expressed her gratitude and went home to Gojō [twenty kilometers northeast of Shunrinken, in present-day Nara Prefecture]. About twenty days later, she came to see me again. She said she recovered from the pain of the beriberi after taking my medicine, and was hoping to be treated for breast cancer. On examining her, I found that indeed, she no longer had beriberi, but now there were signs of asthma. [The asthma was causing her to cough.] This had to be alleviated before she received treatment for breast cancer. I wrote two prescriptions, for *Senkin-soshiin* and *Nanrogan* [herbal remedies], and admitted her to my hospital. After taking the medicines for more than twenty days, every complication was relieved. Thus, the time had come to treat her breast cancer.

After *Mafutsusan* . . .

A vertical incision 7.5 centimeters in length was made over the tumor with a scalpel. The large amount of bleeding from the incision was stopped manually. I inserted my left index finger into the incision to probe the tumor, which was firmly adhered to the surrounding tissues. I separated the tumor from the tissues with the fingers of both hands. Nerves and muscles were cut with the scalpel and a pair of scissors. Bleeding from the vessels was stopped manually.

The tumor was separated from the tissues and excised. The incision was rinsed with shōchū [distilled liquor], and balsam ointment was applied inside. The skin was sutured. Treatment for the incision was the same as for injuries. She was given *kan-yu* [cloudy water in which rice has been washed] for rehydration, *Kanzōshashintō* [a versatile herbal remedy that is still in use today – for anorexia, digestive organ failure, psychic disturbances, sleep disturbances, and the feeling of something stuck in the throat] to facilitate a smooth recovery from general anesthesia, and a bowl of rice porridge.

Her consciousness gradually returned, and she came to realize what had happened. She was surprised to see the incision, and cried, "Where is the tumor? It's gone! I'm very happy. I was never aware of the operation and felt no pain. The tumor has disappeared." I said, persuasively, "Although the tumor was excised without complications, the incision is not yet healed, and your energy hasn't been restored. Rest at my hospital. I want to take care of you daily, by examining you, prescribing medicine, and applying ointments to the wound." She stayed at the hospital at least twenty days. The wound healed completely, and she recovered her usual vitality. Then she went home.

I tried to treat breast cancer before. When I explained my method of surgery to potential patients, they all ran away from the hospital in fear. This woman, however, was different. She entrusted me with her life by allowing me to conduct the operation.

Subsequently, I was able to dispel longstanding doubts about the surgical treatment of breast cancer. To convince my colleagues, I drew illustrations and described the case.

Matsuki learned in 2018 (by deciphering *Seishūidan*, in which Hanaoka describes Kan's postoperative course) that Kan got an infection eight days after surgery. The incision site and her left arm were inflamed and swollen, and she had a fever. She recovered by means of a Hanaoka herbal remedy.

~

Nyūgan Chiken-roku (*A Surgical Experience with Breast Cancer*), the above case report on Kan's operation, was misunderstood until Matsuki began studying the original handwritten document. The confusion started with Shūzō Kure, a medical historian and professor of psychiatry, and the author of the 1923 "bible" on Hanaoka, *Seishū Hanaoka and His Surgery*.

First of all, he wrongly assumed that the report, which is in Chinese, is in Hanaoka's handwriting. Kure revered Hanaoka, so perhaps to give his hero nice writing, he corrected mistakes in some characters, and left out other incorrect characters altogether, when he reproduced it for his book. He also put in illustrations that he said were in the original. But they were not. (The original manuscript included five illustrations that were lost but later found by Matsuki.)

The errors continued via a modern Japanese translation that was based on Kure's version. Naturally, Japanese writers used the Japanese edition as source material – and just like that, the errors developed a life of their own. The handwritten manuscript conundrum is explored further in chapter 10.

The Chinese written language, Japan's first writing and the basis for the alphabet developed later for Japanese, had arrived in the fifth century. Hanaoka knew it very well, so he wouldn't have made the simple mistakes that Kure corrected. Someone with a weak grasp of the Chinese used for the subject of medicine must have recorded the case report for him. Matsuki, who can read old Chinese, compared it to a known sample of Hanaoka's writing: a Certificate of Completion of medical training that he awarded to a Shunrinken student in 1816. The documents appear to have been written by two different people. The probable scenario is that Hanaoka dictated the report to one of his assistants.

Kure got the year wrong too. He thought the operation happened in 1805, not 1804. After Matsuki determined that the report says it took place about forty days after her initial examination, in early September 1804, he searched for her date of death. He found it in March 1971 at the Kōmidōji

Temple in Gojō: the notice says the "Mother of Rihei Aiya" died on February 26, 1805. Once and for all, surgery in October 1805 was ruled out. ("Aiya" was the name of her son Rihei's shop, a typical source of last names.)

The death notice also revealed that Kan died just four and a half months after her operation. *Medical Lectures by Master Seishū Hanaoka*, written by a Shunrinken student, gives this account:

> The mother of someone from Gojō was suffering from breast cancer. The tumor was like a plum seed at the first examination, and a tumor in the axilla [armpit] was palpable. The breast tumor was excised within five hours of an anesthetic administration. The excised tumor weighed about 25 grams.

The presence of a tumor in the axilla means the breast cancer had metastasized. Her prognosis couldn't have been predicted because metastasis was not yet a well understood concept. Later, in 1811, Hanaoka came to realize that breast cancer was likely to recur postoperatively when metastasis to the axillar lymph nodes (among other signs) had been observed. From then on, he adopted stricter criteria for surgery, and taught this to his students.

Kan's death isn't mentioned in the case report. It could be that Hanaoka lost his enthusiasm for completing it when he heard the news. She was his first anesthetized patient – her operation marked the beginning of his work treating breast cancer – so he must have been devastated. Wondering if his procedures had somehow contributed to her death, he turned his attention to a thorough reassessment. He didn't operate again that year (his second breast cancer operation had been on January 6, 1805, a month and a half before Kan died), and he closed down the school.

When the analysis revealed that his procedures were not to blame, he reopened the school and resumed his surgical practice. The next two operations were on April 8 and June 12, 1806. (There was one other long gap between operations: the entire year of 1826, when Hanaoka was 65/66. He wrote a letter to his brother Rokujō around that time saying he was in poor health – so that's probably the explanation for the gap.)

~

Rather than coming up with a word for anesthesia, Hanaoka was content to explain how Kan responded to *Mafutsusan*. A possible reason he didn't name it: when something is invented for a specific purpose – in this case, freedom from surgical trauma – it may not be a concept yet. If no concept, then nothing to name. The invention is simply serving the purpose. The concept of anesthesia came later, and it was called *masui* (details in chapter 12).

Hanaoka used seventeen Chinese characters to describe Kan's reaction that day. This is the translation:

On the morning of October 13, she took my *Mafutsusan.*
A while later she became drowsy and lost consciousness.
Her whole body was numbed, and she felt no pain.

9. Then the People Come

The ultimate goal of medicine is to maintain uninterrupted circulation of the vital components – energy, blood, and water – throughout the body, thereby helping the patient live out his or her natural lifespan (KATSUBUTSU-KYURI).

– Seishū Hanaoka's motto

Changes were in the air. The role of Japanese surgeons had been more or less limited to treating wounds from accidents and sword fights. Not anymore. Rumors *really* started flying after Hanaoka's record eight breast cancer operations in 1808; student enrollment increased dramatically in 1809 as a result, despite the high cost of tuition. Some hoped to earn the right to use *Mafutsusan*. Others came just for the honor of being a Shunrinken student.

Giesecke & Matsuki

> In all, he trained about 1,070 doctors in the school. In addition, he did research in antisepsis, was involved in community leadership, wrote poetry and became a skilled calligrapher. . . . His innovative practices of medicine, anesthesia and surgery have earned him the title of "Great Master of Medicine."

The Epitaph

Neighbors were surprised at first and then denied you, but finally, they became devoted to you and praised you as a second Kada.

Chinese surgeon Huà Tuó (late second century AD), "Kada" in Japan, developed and used an anesthetic called *Mafeisan* in Chinese and *Mafutsusan* in Japanese. His records were lost or destroyed, and though many have tried, no one has been able to work out what the formula was. Kada practiced surgery despite the Confucian belief that it is a form of mutilation; when he died (he was executed for refusing to be the personal doctor of a brutal dictator), surgery was put on hold in China. Hanaoka selected the name *Mafutsusan* to honor the man who demonstrated that anesthesia was possible.

The Mayaku Kō Preface on Kada

Why are people praising him as a doctor with divine skill? Is it not for the following reason? First, he gave the patient *Mafeisan* with wine. He incised the abdomen or the back and removed the lesion after the patient lost consciousness. If disease festered deep in the stomach or intestines, the abdomen was opened for excision and cleansing. After the skin was sutured, topical ointment was applied. His treatment seemed strange and suspicious, but it wasn't impossible. . . . *Mafeisan* was a great invention, but its existence remains a great mystery.

SHUNRINKEN HOSPITAL

The hospital was founded by Seishū's father, Naomichi (also called Jikidō) Hanaoka. Since the building was small, squeezing in the extra patients post-*Mafutsusan* was difficult. Seishū was exactly where he wanted to be:

> Ever since I took over my father's profession more than twenty years ago, I have been practicing medicine. I owe my deceased father a debt of gratitude for what I am today. Many people suffering from protracted diseases come and see me, despite living a thousand miles away.

> I was destined to be a medical doctor. Since I have become one, I think I deserve lashes in public if I fail to cure the curable. How can I forget my duty for even a day?

Diseases that doctors considered hopeless were cured by his innovations. And since he stayed committed to safety, surgical complications were few and far between during his three decades of operations – from 1804 until his death in 1835, just short of his 75th birthday – over a hundred and forty of which were for breast cancer.

He also handled other forms of cancer, traumatic injuries, fractures, necrotic bones, and amputations.

In 1810, the powdered form of *Mafutsusan* was discontinued because it tended to cause nausea and vomiting. From then on, it was prepared as a decoction ("from cooking"), a process whereby an essence (in this case, of a blend of herbs) is extracted with boiling water. The result was consumed as a warm drink. This change, as well as herbal remedies given preoperatively, improved the situation. It was sometimes referred to as *Mafutsutō* after that because the suffix *tō* means decoction (*san* means powder). *Tsūsensan*, yet another name, and one that is often seen in print, was suggested by the doctor husband of Hanaoka's daughter Kame. But the current thinking is to stick with *Mafutsusan*, the original name, because Hanaoka himself chose it, and because that's what he and most of his students called it.

The Epitaph

> Taking the condition of the patient into consideration, you made a decoction of *Mafutsusan*, or *Tsūsensan*, and then treated the disease by excising the affected site. You cured thousands of people, most frequently those with breast cancer.

A Treatise on Mafutsutō, a ten-page set of specific instructions – the first such details – was written in 1839 by Hajime Matsuoka, a student of one of Hanaoka's top students. It explains contraindications, potential dangers, remedies for vomiting, signs for when to begin the operation, postoperative care, and dosage. An adult dose was 10.5 grams boiled in 360 milliliters of water, to make a decoction of approximately 250 milliliters. Half to three-quarters of it was given to patients between the ages of 11 and 15, and a quarter to a half to those between 5 and 10. It wasn't considered safe for children under 5, so they were operated on without sedation.

While nausea/vomiting was the most common issue with *Mafutsusan*, also on record are reactions such as unsatisfactory induction, acute exophthalmos (bulging of the eye out of the orbit), and death during the procedure.

Knowing that surgery is riskier, especially under general anesthesia, if the patient's overall condition is subpar, Hanaoka would first prescribe treatment as needed. On operation day, he instructed patients to eat only two-thirds of their usual breakfast. Typically, an adult was anesthetized within two hours. If the criteria – dilated pupils, flushed face, rapid breathing and pulse, dry lips and tongue, and a frequent urge to urinate one hour later – were met, the time for surgery had arrived.

Infections were common because antisepsis wasn't completely understood yet in Japan (or anywhere). The hands of the surgeon and assistants were not disinfected, and surgical instruments were washed in well water alone. Still, Hanaoka was careful to remove blood coagulants and foreign bodies, and he would wash the wound with shōchū (distilled liquor) or sake (fermented liquor) applied with a syringe. Depending on how deep it was, a drain for discharging blood and purulent matter would be inserted.

He sewed incisions back together using thread made of linen (coarse for large wounds; fine for small ones), and both straight and curved needles. Rose water or palm oil was applied to the perimeter of the wound, which was covered with three sheets of cotton gauze soaked in balsam and egg white, followed by three additional sheets of gauze soaked in vinegar. An assortment of healing ointments was used for treating infections.

Patients were served green tea and green bean soup when they woke up.

Matsuki spent many, many years identifying the survival times of thirty-three of Hanaoka's breast cancer surgical patients (Kan being one of them). It took so long because of how complicated it was to find, then to get permission to examine, the death notices. (Today, laws to protect privacy are so strict that this kind of study has become impossible.) He has recently determined that the average length of time the thirty-three women lived after surgery was about four and a third years. Several of them had traveled a great distance as a last resort, with cancer that was likely at an advanced stage, so this is considered to be an outstanding result.

Shunrinken breast cancer records say the cancer recurred in about seven percent of the more than a hundred and forty patients on whom Hanaoka operated. Another outstanding result. He gained a better understanding of the warning signs for postoperative recurrences of breast cancer in 1811, as noted in chapter 8. Knowledge of this is brand-new; Matsuki finished deciphering *Fujin-nyūronyoku* (*A Handbook on Women's Breast Diseases*), a collection of Hanaoka's lectures, in the nick of time for its contents to be included in this book.

The two-volume handbook was written and illustrated by Shunrinken student Ryōkei Amenomori. As the legends indicate, two illustrations portray women under the influence of Hanaoka's anesthetic (called *Mafutsutō* here) and in the midst of breast cancer surgery. In one, surgery is about to begin; in the other, it's underway and blood is cascading down the left side of the patient. Amenomori's text describes the operations in vivid detail. These are the earliest known illustrations of Hanaoka-style surgery that show the whole patient, not just the surgical site. They therefore could be the first illustrations of people under general anesthesia in the world.

Amenomori entered Shunrinken in 1813. The program normally took two to three years, so he probably created this valuable record in the mid-1810s. The wording is mostly his, but there are also traces of dictation: the order of some of the Chinese characters follows oral expression. It was replicated – text as well as illustrations – in 1826 by Sazen Inoue, a student of Amenomori. The original manuscript and the first volume of the replica were later lost. What remains is Inoue's second volume, which is what Matsuki had the opportunity to study. Here's what he says about how it fell into his hands:

> Ten years ago I became acquainted with Dr. Masataka Amenomori (he is 88 now), who practices 80 kilometers north of Kyoto. He had a manuscript by Ryōkei Amenomori, a distant relative, but he didn't understand it. He gave me a copy to interpret because I'm a vigorous researcher of Hanaoka.
>
> It has taken me ten years to understand the contents. This is partly because I had to learn the details of Hanaoka's style of treating breast diseases and breast cancer, and partly because there were no previous studies on the subject. Of course, the illustrations themselves are easy to understand, but as a medical historian I also had to understand the surrounding descriptions.

This document, a window to a remarkable moment in history, is housed in the Kannon Museum in Nagahama, Japan.

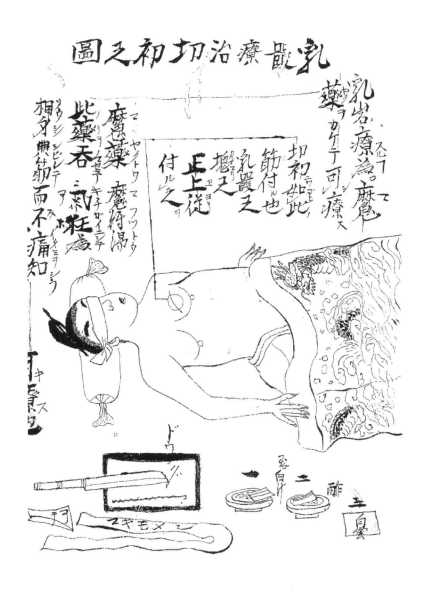

A patient under the influence,
just before breast cancer surgery

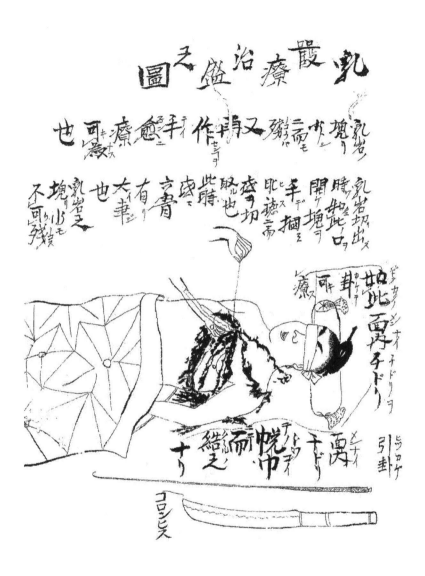

Another patient; she is in the middle of surgery
Note the bleeding from the incision site

SHUNRINKEN MEDICAL SCHOOL

Hanaoka was a dedicated educator. He taught traditional and modern medicine at the medical school he himself founded. Just a few students at a time, and only men because women weren't attending medical school yet. One Shunrinken student reported that the program was excellent, efficient, and could be finished in a hundred days.

The duration of study varied, however, because Hanaoka only gave licenses to those he felt had earned it – that is, those who took personal responsibility for their education. He considered natural ability as well when determining if someone was eligible for graduation. He believed that without it, the individual would forever be clumsy at the art of surgery.

From an 1816 Medical License

> I instructed you earnestly and kindly for a long period of time in the medical arts handed down in my family. Whether or not you have mastered them depends entirely on you. Continue to study hard without laziness. And remember, the secret arts should never be given away, not even to your friends.

The Epitaph

> You taught your art to your students, and talented doctors were produced.

Medical School Rules

- Understand that the most important thing is to learn the practice of medicine.

- Be kind and polite to the patients.

- Work hard from eight to twelve hours every day.

- Do not handle any of the secret herbal formulas.

- Do not reproduce the secret manuscripts before finishing your surgical training.

- If you break the previous rule, your copy will be confiscated.

- Do not behave discourteously to your seniors or to Seishū and his family.

- Do not wander around, argue, or fight in the neighborhood.

- Do not sexually harass women.

- Sweep and scrub the rooms.

TWO OTHER LOCATIONS

Wakayama

In 1802, Hanaoka attained the status of samurai – the military elite in pre-industrial Japan – and was given the privilege of wearing swords (see portrait on page 3). He advanced to the lowest rank of feudal surgeon in 1813, and then was promoted a step higher in 1819. In 1833, two years before he died, he was promoted again. Feudal surgeons worked in the capital city of the estate. (Regular doctors were called village or town practitioners.) There were many ranks; the highest took care of the lord and his family. These positions were usually hereditary, but some, like Hanaoka, were hired for their abilities and accomplishments.

He accepted the job in Wakayama on the condition that they allow him to stay in his village two weeks a month. He opened a small Shunrinken branch in a Wakayama inn.

Osaka

Rokujō Hanaoka, like his brother Seishū, studied liberal arts, and traditional and modern medicine, in Kyoto. In 1816, he established a branch of Shunrinken in Osaka called Gassuidō. Rokujō got sick in late 1826 (when Seishū was also sick), came home to Hirayama, and died in April 1827.

10. Not by the Book

Your great achievement is a divine blessing. I heard that because of your success, some of your students are trying to persuade you to publish. This is reasonable. If you have any plans for publication, please let me know.

– Keizan Asakura (1755-1818), doctor in Kyoto
From an 1808 letter to his friend Seishū

The above encouragement notwithstanding, Hanaoka had no such plans because he equated medical books with predetermined diagnoses and treatment. The way he saw it, applying textbook advice across the board could potentially do harm. If the patient's uniqueness wasn't properly assessed, he was afraid the doctor might choose the wrong medication or dose. Or the right medication/dose, but at the wrong time. In other words, instead of practicing medicine by the book, he thought his response to every patient and student should be creative, spontaneous, and above all, personal.

Two other reasons for not bothering to publish: he had plenty of patients and students as it was, and he was praised by medical leaders when he was still a mere village practitioner. His work was therefore already known and respected.

From a Matsuki abstract

> Seishū Hanaoka chose not to publish medical text-books, in part because of the discrepancy he saw between standardized written advice and the individual treatment patients actually require. He would often say, "My medical skill is a spontaneous response of my hands to what comes into my head, so it's difficult to express this process in words." Instead, his writings are handwritten manuscripts. In *Yōkashinsho* (*Essential Procedures for Traumatic Injuries*), the most widely circulated one, Hanaoka describes his style of surgery and how it developed. The manuscript was repeatedly copied for more than half a century, during which time both the title and contents changed and evolved. Nineteen titles with similar contents have been found; *Hanaoka Seishū Sensei Kōju*, dated 1807, is the earliest.

In September 1861, during a time when Hanaoka's son Roshū was in charge of Shunrinken, student Jikei Satō compiled *The List of Hanaoka's Manuscripts*.

From Satō's preface

> Seishū did not accept any suggestions to publish because he thought books were of no use. However, the only way to master the essence of his medicine is through his writings, so we cannot deny their value. Despite his disdain for publishing, Seishū dictated a considerable amount of information to his students.

The manuscripts were copied frequently, and circulated widely, so there is confusion between different titles with the same contents and the same title with different contents. Also, having multiple copies has resulted in a number of mistakes in characters and phrases, making them difficult to understand. This is regrettable. I have been trying to correct the mistakes for a long time.

As Matsuki's abstract and Satō's preface point out, the trouble with handwritten copies of copies is that as time goes by, they are less and less like the original.

~

Kōmō-gekashū (*Collected Writings on Dutch Surgery*) is the earliest document in Hanaoka's own handwriting. It is dated February 26, 1784: the middle of his medical school years. The manuscript describes surgical pathology, wound treatment, a variety of ointments and prescriptions, and 308 Dutch words and their Japanese translations. He probably used it as a textbook.

Another manuscript, *Rare Diseases Treated by Hanaoka*, was written by his students around 1840. There are several copies; one is housed in the Wood Library-Museum (WLM) of Anesthesiology in Schaumburg, Illinois:

Each one is a little different because each was done by hand. The WLM has acquired one of these copies for its rare book collection. The book consists of 52 pages of hand-drawn illustrations with sparse text written in Japanese. Forty-six are in color and the remainders are black and white. The green silk cover is hand-stitched to bind the pages together, and the whole is preserved in a green silk slipcover.

~

The "East meets West" style of medical care and education at Shunrinken faded temporarily after Hanaoka's death, due to the shift in nineteenth century Japan away from traditional medicine, and because his individualized approach depended on his physical presence. Once he was gone, his followers had only unstable handwritten manuscripts to consult.

But before that day arrived, Hanaoka trained many like-minded doctors. Two students, Genchō Honma (1804-1872) and Gendai Kamata (1794-1854), followed closely in Hanaoka's footsteps, and even built on his techniques.

Also, they published.

Genchō Honma entered Shunrinken in March 1827. He published the ten-volume *Secret Records of Surgery* in 1847 and the five-volume *Secret Records of Surgery: Continued* in 1859. During the twelve years between his books, Honma became a skilled surgeon, able to do two procedures previously beyond his reach: a leg amputation above the knee and a tongue tumor excision. He finally succeeded because he mastered how to suture blood vessels to control the bleeding. Hanaoka had tried unsuccessfully to control bleeding by suturing vessels to the surrounding tissues.

An illustration in *Continued* shows the leg amputation of 35-year-old Tatsuzō Okabe, a man who'd been suffering from gangrene for ten years. Okabe was under the influence of *Mafutsusan* on April 5, 1857, when Honma amputated his right leg. This was the first amputation above the knee with anesthesia in Japan.

Concerned about all the confusion over the manuscripts, he identified, in 1850, twenty-one of the most authentic and essential ones. His compilation has been extremely helpful to medical historians studying Hanaoka.

To trace advances in breast cancer surgery in the first half of the nineteenth century in Japan, Matsuki compared Hanaoka's tumor excisions in 1804-15 with those of Honma in 1830-50. He found that their operative methods, ointments, and postoperative medications were similar, but that Honma provided much more careful incisional wound treatment.

Gendai Kamata entered Shunrinken in March 1812 and, like Honma, became a skilled surgeon. He published *Illustrations of Surgical Cases* in 1840, and the ten-volume *Surgical Cases* in 1851. *A Treatise on Mafutsutō*, discussed in chapter 9, is in the latter book; its author was Kamata's student. One of Kamata's contributions to medicine is a technique to tighten the base of a tumor using two sticks of bamboo. This made the excision easier, and also reduced the bleeding. Another is a technique to insert a surgical instrument called a trocar into the abdominal cavity to drain ascites (abnormal accumulation of fluid). Hanaoka tried to puncture a bladder with a trocar but never an abdominal cavity.

Kamata followed his teacher's approach to life: he wasn't interested in fame or money, and didn't differentiate between his rich and poor patients. Impressed by all of this, and by Kamata's skills, Hanaoka made him a scroll that included a Chinese poem he had written (in his later years, he designed and created scrolls for his best students).

The words of the poem capture the essence of Hanaoka's philosophy:

> *By my bamboo thatch in desolation, wild fowl warble;*
> *The scenery satisfies me in this village so humble.*
> *I always intend only to cure the incurable, and*
> *Eschew a life of fleet steeds and feather apparel.*

In the original Chinese version, each line has seven characters and the sound *'n* at the end of the first, second, and fourth lines. For the English translation, Matsuki tried to keep it to seven words per line, but that wasn't possible without losing meaning. He settled on nine, with the condition that the end of the first, second, and fourth lines end with the same sound, which he decided would be *'l*.

Hanaoka's scrolls are not only beautiful calligraphy, they are also his perspectives, his thoughts, his ideas. They mean a great deal more than books.

11. A Secret Is Revealed

*Your name is well known here . . . I am deeply
impressed by your accomplishments.*

– Genpaku Sugita (1733-1817), feudal surgeon
From his 1812 letter to Hanaoka requesting
the formula for *Mafutsusan*

She gradually became unconscious, and then lost awareness.

– Ryūkei Sugita (1786-1845), feudal surgeon
and Genpaku's son
On his use of *Mafutsusan* for breast cancer surgery in 1813

Because of a chance connection to Hanaoka through a medical student, Genpaku Sugita and his son Ryūkei are a part of the *Mafutsusan* story. Genpaku (for the sake of clarity, the first names of father and son are used here) was one of the men who translated an anatomy book after observing the dissection of a beheaded convict (chapter 3). The student, Juntatsu Miyakawa, studied at Shunrinken from 1806 to 1808, then transferred to Genpaku's medical school, where he spoke of Hanaoka's surgical magic. Genpaku was thrilled. Meeting Miyakawa, who had himself performed breast cancer surgery with *Mafutsusan*, was giving him a once-in-a-lifetime chance to learn more about the person responsible for the new anesthetic. He decided to request the formula:

May 4, 1812

Dear Zuiken Hanaoka [another of Seishū's names; it was given to the oldest son of each generation],

I have not yet had the honor of making your acquaintance, but please permit me to address a letter to you. The weather is getting milder, and I am happy to hear that you are in the best of health. Your name is well known here in Edo. Since last year, Juntatsu Miyakawa, previously a student at your school, has been studying at mine; he said you have worked hard at your practice for many years. I am deeply impressed by your accomplishments.

For several generations, my forefathers have served in the Obama Domain [feudal estate based in the port city of Obama, in present-day Fukui Prefecture] as feudal surgeons, and I, as a feudal surgeon too, have been trying to offer better medical care for a long time. Unfortunately, my results haven't been favorable. Time passes and my humble self will be 80 soon; I regret that I shall die in obscurity.

When I have questions connected to my specialty, I am unable to find a surgeon who can answer them. While I knew your name, I haven't had a chance to communicate with you, so it is fortunate that Miyakawa came here to talk about your excellent practice of medicine.

As you are aware, many patients would be cured by surgery. Most of them, however, are very apprehensive of the pain; they are like timid nobles, unable to tolerate it. I know they need treatment, but regrettably, I cannot provide them with it. Because I am of an advanced age, I would like to ask you to extend a favor to my sons. When they seek your advice by epistle, please forgive them for doing so.

I heard that Juntatsu has addressed a letter to you, so I am writing this in haste. I would greatly appreciate it if you include my name among your acquaintances.

Respectfully,
Genpaku Sugita

Having translated part of *Heelkundige Onderwyzingen* (*Surgical Education*), the 1776 Dutch edition of a surgery book by Lorenz Heister, Genpaku and Ryūkei were familiar with the basics of surgery in the western world. But they couldn't find something in the book: how those surgeons dealt with pain. Why was nothing there? Because nothing was done! Genpaku wanted to do more than treat wounds, but he couldn't bear to see his patients writhing in agony. Though he was somewhat ashamed of this decision, he knew that was where he had to draw the line.

Until he met Miyakawa. He thought that perhaps his new student could provide the link to blessed pain relief. Requesting the formula was a bold move, despite being more famous than Hanaoka, because of the Japanese tradition of secrecy. Keeping methods secret was standard practice in schools of art such as judō, karate, kendō, floral art, and the tea ceremony. The medical world was no exception, so at that time, surgeons educated at Shunrinken were the only ones anesthetizing their patients.

Hanaoka's manuscripts describe his techniques, diagnoses, prescriptions, specialties, and postoperative care. Many were available to his students; in fact, they were instrumental in spreading his methods throughout the country. As for the formulas, the traditional blends were public knowledge, but while the *ingredients* of the newly-developed prescription were public, the ratios, especially that of *Datura* to *Aconitum*, were closely guarded.

Preventing anesthesia-related injuries was the reason for the secrecy. For one thing, the airway is easily blocked under general anesthesia, and for another, *Mafutsusan* had a narrow safety margin due to the inclusion of *Datura* and *Aconitum*. Hanaoka did teach students how to prepare and use it, but only those with character traits necessary to handle it properly. Chloroform's path is one example of what can happen when powerful drugs are readily accessible. It began as an anesthetic in 1847, rapidly spread worldwide, and ended up causing thousands of deaths.

~

Hanaoka was convinced. Genpaku and Ryūkei had virtuous reputations, so there was no reason to say no to this (implied) request for *Mafutsusan*. He gave them the formula.

The following year, in September 1813, Genpaku examined a woman with breast cancer and found a tumor the size of a teacup in her right breast. Her skin hadn't changed color, the tumor was not adhered to the wall of her chest, and she was in pain only occasionally, so he was confident a surgical excision would cure her. Later that month, using *Mafutsusan*, Ryūkei performed the operation. The woman's name, age, and how long she lived are not known. *Ryō Nyūgan Ki* (*A Record of Breast Cancer Treatment*) is his account:

Ryūkei's Mafutsusan Experience

> Genpaku, my father, explained to her, "If the tumor is not excised, the cancer will advance further and you will suffer greatly. The excision is not to be feared, but

it isn't easy to do. We cannot even predict our lives for today. If there is a grave complication during surgery, the surgeon is responsible. Please discuss this with your family." She listened and then went home. About ten days later, she and her husband requested surgery, even if the worst were to happen. Genpaku accepted their request, and asked me to conduct the operation because he thought he was too old.

On September 16, 1813, I gave the woman the anesthetic and prepared the instruments. She gradually became unconscious, and then lost awareness. A cruciform incision was made on her right breast, 5 centimeters long and 7 centimeters across. Much blood loss occurred during the procedure to remove the tumor and a small amount of tissue around it. The deep part of the wound was cleansed using cotton soaked in shōchū. An ointment was applied inside the wound, which was then covered with cotton soaked in balm. A pressure bandage was placed on top. She recovered from anesthesia six hours later, and was completely cured in a month.

Seishū Hanaoka read in *Miscellaneous Travel Notes* that breast cancer was excised surgically in western countries [without anesthesia, as explained in chapter 4; the book came out in 1764, before there was such a thing]. This prompted him to operate on breast cancer patients by means of his own invention. Juntatsu Miyakawa, who was once a student of Hanaoka, recently enrolled in Genpaku's medical school. He has operated successfully on several patients with breast cancer.

Having a deep respect for Hanaoka's philosophy from afar, and observing Miyakawa's skills up close, I added western knowledge to theirs and achieved success.

Such a story is possible only in this time of peace. I am thankful for the wonders of life, and I want to share my overwhelming joy with others.

~

Miscellaneous Travel Notes (*Man-yū Zakki*) is the book, as noted in chapter 4, that played a big part in Hanaoka's decision to pursue breast cancer surgery. It also inspired him to collect and study "extra-traditional" (newly developed) herbal prescriptions. The result: he found a way to transport his surgical patients into a blissful state of unawareness and painlessness.

12. Going Dutch

Mafutsusan is never coming back because . . .

- *It took one to two hours to induce anesthesia.*
- *Its depth and duration were very difficult to control.*
- *There was no way to wake the patient up early.*
- *Even the decocted version sometimes caused vomiting.*
- *It was administered orally, which limited its indication.*
- *It couldn't be given to abdominal patients.*
- *The safety margin was narrow because it contained Datura and Aconitum.*

– A. Matsuki
June 3, 2016, email to E. Bunker

In 1954, in recognition of his phenomenal contributions to the art of surgery, Seishū Hanaoka was inducted into the Hall of Fame of the International College of Surgeons in Chicago, Illinois. To say the least, he made excellent use of the science and the resources that were available in his day. But in the 1850s, two decades after his death, everything began to shift. *Mafutsusan* was on its way out, and chloroform was taking its place.

News about the anesthesia discoveries in the West in the 1840s initially trickled in via the Dutch Factory, but all that changed when Japan's doors were forced open a few years later (recounted in chapter 3). Chloroform was fast and reliable, critical in emergency situations like the battlefields of the Boshin War – the 1868-69 civil war that was triggered by the humiliation of the forced opening – so Japanese doctors welcomed the anesthetic. *Kaitai Shinsho*, the 1774 anatomy book translated by Genpaku Sugita and colleagues, and the success of the smallpox vaccine in 1849, also contributed to the tilt toward modern western medicine. (Traditional, modern, and various combinations of the two are all practiced freely today. Those who choose to specialize in traditional medicine are certified by the Japanese Society of Oriental Medicine.)

Most of the world got ahold of ether before chloroform. By happenstance, the order was reversed in Japan. The Japanese-with-a-dash-of-Dutch story of the switch to chloroform in a moment, but first . . .

Chloroform, or trichloromethane, is a volatile (evaporates easily) liquid chemical compound that's approximately forty times sweeter than sugar. The formula is $CHCl_3$. It was once a common ingredient in cough syrups, pain relievers, and sedatives. It's still in use in the production of pesticides and dyes, and as a solvent in the pharmaceutical industry: chloroform extracts alkaloids from plants, such as morphine from poppies and scopolamine from *Datura*. Shades of *Mafutsusan*.

The compound was synthesized independently in 1831 by scientists in three different countries: Samuel Guthrie of the United States, Eugène Soubeiran of France, and Justus von Liebig of Germany. Its anesthetic and toxic effect on animals was described in March 1847.

Eight months later, on the evening of November 4, 1847, at a dinner party in Edinburgh, Scotland, obstetrician James Y. Simpson and two assistants inhaled chloroform fumes as an experiment. They were hoping to find a pain-relief method for childbirth. An acquaintance familiar with the compound, a doctor named David Waldie, had told Simpson that it could be just the thing he was looking for. Simpson had already investigated ether, newly recognized as an effective anesthetic, but he wasn't satisfied. He wanted something less unpleasant to inhale, more potent, and that didn't explode, as ether did, when a flame was nearby. Suffice it to say, the men woke up in the morning under the furniture. Mrs. Simpson's niece also joined in the fun; as the chloroform took hold, she came to the conclusion that she was a flying angel.

Simpson and chloroform became overnight sensations. Waldie – *whose idea it was* – is a mere footnote of history.

It was sprinkled onto a sponge or a cloth, then the vapor was inhaled. The speed of induction was impressive, but this dense colorless liquid turned out to be riskier than originally thought, and administering it required skills that were often missing due to the headlong rush to use it. There was a fine line between the correct dose – and one that wasn't correct. The high number of fatalities was well publicized, and some potential surgical patients, fearing death, opted for the pain. A 15-year-old girl died eleven weeks after its first use. People died from liver failure shortly after their operations. But still, it was the anesthetic of choice practically everywhere (it never overtook ether in the United States, however).

Queen Victoria inhaled a bit of chloroform from a handkerchief during the birth of her eighth child, Prince Leopold, in 1853, and of her ninth, Princess Beatrice, in 1857. Enough to take the edge off, without loss of awareness. Anesthesia with childbirth was hardly commonplace, so this news was alarming. How could her doctor have allowed it? But it had been her decision, and her example eventually made it fashionable to inhale chloroform when giving birth.

~

Ether and nitrous oxide got their start as recreational drugs. "Ether frolics" and "laughing gas parties" were springboards to inhalation anesthesia once it was evident that when people got hurt at these events, they felt no pain.

- January 1842: first recorded use of inhalation anesthesia. Medical student William E. Clarke administered ether to "Miss Hobbie," a classmate's sister, and dentist Elijah Pope pulled out her tooth. Rochester, NY.

- March 30, 1842: second use. General practitioner Crawford W. Long excised two tumors from James Venable's neck after administering ether. Jefferson, GA.

- December 11, 1844: first use of nitrous oxide for a surgical procedure. Dentist Horace Wells *put himself under*; friend and fellow dentist John M. Riggs then extracted a bothersome wisdom tooth. (While Dec. 11 is the official day, several people, including Wells himself, said it was early November and/or the fall.) Hartford, CT.

- October 16, 1846: first successful public demonstration that was witnessed by the U.S. medical establishment. Surgeon John C. Warren performed a neck tumor excision on Gilbert Abbott with ether administered by dentist William T. G. Morton, who learned about ether and nitrous oxide from Wells and scientist Charles T. Jackson. Massachusetts General Hospital, Boston, MA.

Realization struck Clarke, Long, and Wells when they saw people oblivious to injuries after enjoying ether and nitrous oxide. They got the idea independently of each other, but only Wells spread the news about anesthesia and dared to be the first patient. He wasn't interested in making money from it: "I was desirous that it be as free as the air we breathe."

Because the Warren-Morton operation caught the ear of the establishment, ether was suddenly big news. In a flash, nineteen books were published in Germany. The title of one of them, by Joseph Schlesinger, left little to the imagination: *Die Einathmung des Schwefel-Aethers in ihren Wirkungen auf Menschen und Thiere, besonders als ein Mittel bei chirurgischen Operationen den Schmerz zu umgehen* ("The effects of the inhalation of sulfur-ether on men and animals, especially as a means to circumvent the pain of surgical operations"). The book came out in 1847, was translated into Dutch that year, and arrived in Japan in 1849.

Government translator Seikei Sugita (Ryūkei's son and Genpaku's grandson) translated the Dutch edition into Japanese in 1850.

Ten years later, three Japanese doctors had a memorable encounter with ether in the United States. A delegation had gone there for the ratification of the 1858 Treaty of Amity and Commerce (a.k.a. the Harris Treaty), the second of two U.S. treaties requiring Japan to dismantle its isolationist policies. The seventy-two Japanese visitors traveled around the country, including to the White House, where they met President James Buchanan. The doctors – Hakugen Murayama, Ryūgen Miyazaki, and Dōmin Kawasaki, all trained in traditional Chinese medicine – were given the opportunity to observe an operation at the Gross Clinic in Philadelphia, Pennsylvania. Surgeon Samuel D. Gross removed bladder stones from the patient, using ether administered by Morton, the dentist who demonstrated its effectiveness in Boston fourteen years earlier. An interpreter explained the proceedings.

That day was a revelation to Murayama, Miyazaki, and Kawasaki – they even got to pour ether on their hands and feel the chill as it evaporated – and, in turn, to doctors back home. They were given surgery books, medical instruments, and (of all things) a set of false teeth. Gross' new book *A System of Surgery: Pathological, Diagnostic, Therapeutic and Operative* (1859) was among the gifts. (They couldn't read it, but a Japanese translation of the section on chloroform appeared in 1868 in *Essentials for Amputations* by Motonori Tashiro. This book gave a boost to chloroform's popularity.)

Despite the enlightening American experience had by the three Japanese doctors, ether never caught on in their homeland. The reason, in all likelihood, was that those spreading the word about the western inhalants had only seen an unpurified, and therefore a lot less effective, version of it.

Doctors in Batavia (present-day Jakarta), the capital of the Dutch East Indies, conducted experiments with frogs, fish, birds, rabbits, and dogs when ether got there in 1847. Next, a few people volunteered, but not much happened. One doctor inhaled the fumes himself: he got a headache and felt dizzy. Then, in the early months of 1848, chloroform arrived. It was given to four people facing leg amputations, and finally! Relief from surgical pain. Not entirely, but close enough. German doctor Otto Gottlieb Mohnike, transferred from Batavia to the Dutch Factory in June 1848, departed with the results of these experiments in mind.

Mohnike didn't bring chloroform with him to Japan, and whether or not he used it while there isn't known, but he was the first to convey information about it. (He also administered the smallpox vaccine, in 1849, the time it was finally effective in Japan; there'd been numerous failed attempts.) He was stationed on the island until 1851. Two months after arriving, he said the following about chloroform, the first such comments on record in Japan:

[Chloroform] is excellent for anesthetizing patients to perform surgeries. After pouring several drops of the agent into a tinplate can, the patient covers his mouth with the can to inhale the vapor of the agent. Although he soon feels numbness, he does not lose consciousness. Bearing in mind an adequate inhalation, the patient feels no pain at all during surgery.

When the patient does not recover from numbness after the surgery, a cup of coffee or some decoctions should be given.

Conversely, Mohnike had this to say about ether:

> In some patients, the inhalation of ether not only produces no insensateness but also causes a retardation of incisional wound healing, leading to a serious postoperative result.

After hearing the glowing assessment of chloroform, Japanese officials wanted details. This was less than a year after Simpson and friends' experiment in Scotland, and nothing had been published. At least not in Dutch. But the Dutch edition of the German ether book with the long title had *just* come out – so, like it or not, that's what they got, and that's what was translated. Not only an accomplished translator, Seikei Sugita (1817-1859) was also a feudal surgeon, like his father and grandfather, and a composer of Chinese poetry. His book *Treatises on the Inhalation of Ether* (1850) is the earliest Japanese translation of a western book on anesthesia.

In *Treatises*, Sugita introduced a word for anesthesia – it was still nameless in Japanese – and it caught on. The word, *masui*, comes from *ma* (loss of sensation) and *sui* (loss of consciousness due to drugs or alcohol). In response to the arrival of local anesthesia (cocaine) in the 1880s, qualifying words were added: *kyokusho masui* is local and *zenshin masui* is general. For thirty years, Matsuki was under the impression that

Sugita had invented the word. But then, in 2018, he saw *masui* in a Japanese pediatric textbook (translated from the Dutch), where it was utilized to describe the signs and symptoms of opium use. That book was published in 1845, so when *Treatises* came out in 1850, *masui* was already a word. What Sugita did was find a new meaning for it.

Doctor and poet Oliver Wendell Holmes Sr. named anesthesia for the English-speaking world in 1846.

Sugita scheduled two operations in 1855 with the anesthetic he'd been writing about. Neither was a success because the ether he was using hadn't been purified. The first was to repair a burn scar on the hand of one of his students; after inhaling the vapor, the patient promptly nodded off, only to wake up moments later. They tried again – still nothing, so the procedure went ahead without pain relief. He also tried ether for a breast tumor excision, but the patient remained wide awake. That operation was cancelled. Unlike his father, Sugita never used *Mafutsusan*.

A Dutch doctor with a noteworthy name, Johannes Lijdius Catharinus Pompe van Meerdervoort, was the next person to promote chloroform in Japan. He lived there from 1857 to 1863. Pompe van Meerdervoort (who was actually Dutch, not just "Dutch") is known to have brought chloroform with him, but his use of it wasn't documented.

Initially, he taught medicine and photography at the Naval Training Center in Nagasaki, near Dejima (the Center was a response to the American demands set in motion in 1853 by Commodore Perry, and was run with help from the Netherlands). He later founded a hospital and medical school, where he broke from Japanese tradition by using dissection and autopsy in his anatomy classes. Since cadavers were hard to get in Japan back then, he started off by ordering one from Paris.

One of Pompe van Meerdervoort's students, Ine Kusumoto, was the daughter of the disgraced doctor of Dejima from chapter 3: Philipp Franz von Siebold. Ine stayed with her Japanese mother, Taki, when her father was deported. She went on to become the first female doctor of western medicine in Japan. Another student, Genboku Itō, amputated Yoshijirō Sakuragawa's gangrenous right foot on June 29, 1861, using chloroform supplied by his teacher. This is the first recorded use of it in Japan, thirteen years after Mohnike promoted it there.

Meanwhile, breakthroughs with *Mafutsusan* were still unfolding: the above-the-knee leg amputation by Hanaoka student Genchō Honma had happened four years earlier.

Next for chloroform was the battlefield, with assistance from William Willis of Scotland. This man had a huge impact on the acceptance of the anesthetic in Japan. Appointed to the

British consulate as a doctor in 1862 after applying for overseas service, he treated soldiers wounded in the Boshin War. Any soldiers, no matter what side they were on. The Japanese surgeons who worked with him were impressed by his skills, and by chloroform's speed.

A March 2, 1868, Letter from William Willis to
Sir Harry Smith Parkes, British Minister to Japan

> In twelve cases I found it necessary to perform amputations varying in point of magnitude from removal of part of the hand to amputation of the thigh. I also performed a number of minor operations, such as extracting bullets, removing pieces of dead bone, and opening abscesses. I administered chloroform to all my patients requiring the use of the knife . . . I subsequently learnt that they were greatly encouraged when it came to be known that what I did I effected painlessly.

> I devoted my time to teaching Japanese Doctors and hospital attendants the best methods known to me of treating wounds generally, at the same time considering with them the individual requirements of each case presented to me.

Kenzō Yoshida, after observing Willis, was the second Japanese surgeon to make use of chloroform. In January 1868 he treated a man by the name of Nakamura who had been attempting *hara-kiri* (ritual suicide by cutting open the abdomen and removing the intestines). Yoshida administered the chloroform, squeezed the intestines back in, and then a colleague sewed the man up. Nakamura completely recovered – only to be executed as a criminal shortly thereafter.

Gen-yu Hirota, also after seeing Willis at work, was the third Japanese surgeon to operate with chloroform. He was educated at Gassuidō, the Shunrinken branch run by Seishū's brother Rokujō. Hirota performed amputations for two soldiers in 1868: Taisuke Yoshikawa on April 10 (an arm) and Chozaburo Oda on May 3 (an index finger).

Another road to Japan for the seemingly ideal anesthetic began with a world's fair: the International Exposition of 1867 in Paris. Japan sent lacquerware, ceramics, utensils, and other items to be exhibited. One of the Japanese representatives, surgeon Ryō-un Takamatsu – selected because he spoke English and Dutch – stayed behind to study French and medicine when the fair was over. While in Paris, he learned about chloroform.

A year later, after getting word of his country's civil war, he returned to help the wounded soldiers. Takamatsu arrived home on May 17, 1868. Like Willis, he didn't care what side the soldiers belonged to, which got him into trouble – he did time as a prisoner of war until his captors decided he was behaving as any doctor should. He taught his techniques to his colleagues, and treated about three hundred and eighty men, ninety-seven of whom did not survive.

American surgeons operated with ether during the Mexican-American War (1846-48). By the time the United States' civil war broke out in 1861, seven years before Japan's, chloroform was available too.

~

The use of chloroform and ether declined after the development of safer and more effective anesthetics. Chloroform was found to depress most organs of the body, and to cause sudden cardiac death and liver failure. The Committee on Anesthesia of the American Medical Association said in 1912 that using it as an anesthetic was no longer justified, based on evidence for delayed poisoning. The United States Environmental Protection Agency labeled it a carcinogen in 1976.

In Japan, the first chloroform lawsuit was in May 1912. The plaintiff's claim, which was rejected, concerned a patient who died on June 8, 1911. Chloroform was phased out there around 1965, a century after the controversial anesthetic was given a stamp of approval by "Dutch" doctors stationed on a 2.2-acre fan-shaped "factory" in Nagasaki Bay.

13. What Happens Next

*I was able to dispel longstanding doubts about
the surgical treatment of breast cancer.*

– Seishū Hanaoka

The Dutch Factory

By 1859, there was no longer a need for Dejima. Two centuries of isolation had ended, making Japan's narrow bridge to the land beyond its borders obsolete. A modern Dutch consulate took over the rewritten duties required by modern times. The island was lost to changes in the harbor and the rerouting of a river – but then, in 1922, it was designated a national historic site. A total reconstruction of the one-of-a-kind trading post is gradually becoming a reality.

The Hospital and Medical School

Student enrollment went down in 1835, when Hanaoka died, but it rebounded when his son Roshū took the reins. The first, and only, female student enrolled in 1855. She was the wife of a man by the name of Genshun Fukushima (her first name is unknown). The last breast cancer operations on record there were in 1871. Then, after Hanaoka's grandson Kōdō died in 1882, Shunrinken closed down.

The main building was sold in 1923 to a nearby village. In 1997, it was brought back to Hirayama (now Nishinoyama) and rebuilt; it reopened as Flower Hill Museum ("flower hill" is the definition of *hanaoka*). The site was excavated two years before the building returned, revealing a sophisticated sewer system. The excavation also revealed that the building and grounds were enlarged after October 13, 1804, in order to accommodate the extra patients and students.

The Herbal Anesthetic

An 1899 paper by Gassuidō graduate Kansaku Shindō is the last known record of surgery with *Mafutsusan*. So it overlapped with chloroform for just under forty years. The main reason for the demise of the magnificent invention that benefitted Kan Aiya and many others was the time it took to go into effect, which made it impractical for emergency surgery.

The Doctor

But whereas the anesthetic itself was temporary, the medical practice of the man who created it is timeless. The personal and spontaneous side of Hanaoka-style medicine required his physical presence; still, his influence lives on. He helped pave the way for a perspective that individualizes patient care, that learns from the past while contributing to the future, and that spans from East to West.

You integrated several theories. You used traditional methods but were not trapped. You created new methods, but did not forget tradition. You could cure even rare and intractable diseases that are not described in textbooks.

By going back – figuratively and literally – Seishū Hanaoka was able to go forward. Without that skill, he would never have dreamed up the dazzling fish hook escape, and he would never have sought inspiration in ancient herbal formulas for the sake of painlessness and unawareness in the operating room. Blending traditional and modern medicine is still relevant, for a variety of uses, and is still practiced in Japan.

You were clever and brave from boyhood. You were very active in supporting people in difficult circumstances. You were honest and unaffected, and did not follow fame.

Being remembered may not have mattered to this modest Japanese doctor, but he should be remembered nonetheless. His perspectives on medical care, and on life, transcend time and national boundaries.

TIMELINE

Late second century AD

Chinese doctor Huà Tuó, known as Kada in Japan, develops and uses a general anesthetic. His records have vanished.

754

Blind Chinese Buddhist priest Jian Zhen arrives in Japan to spread Buddhism. He teaches the priests how to use herbs.

984

A book of Chinese medical knowledge, *Ishinhō* (*The Essence of Medicine and Therapeutic Methods*), is published in Japan.

1337

The herbal pain-relief formula *Sō-u-san*, a forerunner to Hanaoka's anesthetic, is described in a Chinese medical book.

1543

The Portuguese arrive.

April 19, 1600

The Dutch arrive.

1614

Christian missionaries are expelled.

By 1639

All westerners except the Dutch have left Japan.

1641

Dejima, a miniature manmade island in Nagasaki Bay known also as the Dutch Factory, becomes a Dutch trading post.

1649-51

German surgeon Caspar Schamberger is stationed on Dejima; he is the first European doctor to serve there.

1672

Datura alba Nees, one of the two principal herbs in Hanaoka's anesthetic, is cultivated in Edo (present-day Tokyo).

1745

Kan Aiya is born.

1754

Tōyō Yamawaki performs the first official human dissection in Japan.

1759

Zōshi (*Explanations of Internal Organs*), Yamawaki's illustrated book about the inside of the human body, is published.

October 23, 1760

Seishū Hanaoka is born.

1764

Man-yū Zakki (*Miscellaneous Travel Notes*) by Dokushōan Nagatomi is published. Two decades later, it inspires Hanaoka to pursue breast cancer surgery, and to collect and study extra-traditional herbal prescriptions.

March 4, 1771

Genpaku Sugita and Ryōtaku Ma-eno witness the dissection of a decapitated criminal in Edo.

1774

Kaitai Shinsho (*New Text on Anatomy*) – a Japanese translation by Sugita, Ma-eno, and others of the Dutch edition of a German anatomy book – is published. Much more accurate than *Zōshi*, it contributes to the acceptance of western medicine.

1782-85

Hanaoka attends medical school in Kyoto.

1795

He returns to Kyoto to study western ointments.

May 1796

Mayaku Kō (*A Treatise on Anesthetics*), a manuscript that describes the evolution of the search for anesthesia in Japan, is written and edited by Shūtei Nakagawa.

1798

Sōkei Gūki by Nan-yō Hara is published. This collection of clinical experiences includes a detailed description of *Datura*.

Summer 1803

Kan notices a tumor in her left breast.

September to September 1803-04

Hanaoka's legs are paralyzed. Experimenting on himself with *Mafutsusan*, his herbal anesthetic, could be the cause.

Early September 1804
Kan begins her consultations with Hanaoka.

October 13, 1804
She has breast cancer surgery – a tumor excision – under the influence of *Mafutsusan*. The first use of general anesthesia for a surgical procedure in recorded history.

January 6, 1805
A second woman has breast cancer surgery with *Mafutsusan*.

February 26, 1805
Kan Aiya dies.

The rest of 1805
Hanaoka closes Shunrinken, his hospital and medical school, in order to turn his attention to sorting out if his surgical procedures contributed to Kan's death.

1806
He reopens Shunrinken after determining that his procedures had nothing to do with it. (Five years later he came to understand why her cancer was beyond help.)

April 8 and June 12, 1806
He performs two more breast cancer operations.

1809
His record eight breast cancer operations in 1808 result in a dramatic increase in student enrollment.

1810

Mafutsusan is administered as a decoction rather than a powder, in an attempt to alleviate a vomiting problem.

May 4, 1812

Feudal surgeon Genpaku Sugita writes to Hanaoka to request the formula for *Mafutsusan*. Hanaoka agrees; this is noteworthy because of the traditional secrecy in medicine.

September 16, 1813

Using *Mafutsusan*, Genpaku's son Ryūkei operates on a breast cancer patient.

Around the mid-1810s

Women having breast cancer surgery under the influence of Hanaoka's anesthetic are illustrated. Possibly the first illustrations of people under general anesthesia in the world.

1816

The earliest known surgery by a student of Hanaoka.

Entire year of 1826

Hanaoka is ill and cannot operate.

October 2, 1835

Seishū Hanaoka dies.

June 1839

A Treatise on Mafutsutō, the first detailed instructions on how to use *Mafutsusan* (*Mafutsutō* is another name for it), is written by a student of a student of Hanaoka.

January 1842

In New York, medical student William E. Clarke administers ether to "Miss Hobbie," a classmate's sister, and dentist Elijah Pope pulls out her tooth. First recorded use of inhalation anesthesia for a surgical procedure; it is Clarke's idea.

December 11, 1844 (possibly a little earlier)

In Connecticut, dentist Horace Wells *puts himself under* with nitrous oxide; friend and fellow dentist John M. Riggs then extracts a bothersome wisdom tooth. First use of laughing gas for a surgical procedure; it is Wells' idea.

1846

Oliver Wendell Holmes Sr. invents the word "anesthesia."

November 4, 1847

In Scotland, obstetrician James Y. Simpson and two assistants, hoping to find a pain-relief method for childbirth, experiment on themselves with chloroform. First recorded inhalation of chloroform; use for surgical procedures/childbirth follows. It is David Waldie's idea (a doctor acquaintance of Simpson).

1848-51

German doctor Otto Gottlieb Mohnike is stationed on Dejima; he is the first in Japan to promote chloroform as an anesthetic.

1850

Seikei Sugita translates the Dutch edition of a book on ether into Japanese. The book, *Treatises on the Inhalation of Ether*, is the first Japanese translation of a western book on anesthesia; it also introduces a Japanese word for anesthesia: *masui*.

April 7, 1853
Queen Victoria inhales chloroform for the birth of her eighth and penultimate child, Prince Leopold.

July 1853
U.S. Commodore Matthew C. Perry arrives in Japan to force the Japanese to end their self-imposed isolation.

March 31, 1854
The Treaty of Kanagawa, the first of two U.S. treaties requiring Japan to dismantle its isolationist policies, is signed.

1857
Johannes Lijdius Catharinus Pompe van Meerdervoort, a doctor from the Netherlands, brings chloroform to Japan.

April 5, 1857
Hanaoka's student Genchō Honma amputates a patient's leg using *Mafutsusan*. First amputation above the knee with anesthesia in Japan.

April 14, 1857
Queen Victoria inhales chloroform for the birth of her ninth and last child, Princess Beatrice.

1859
Dejima, a.k.a. the Dutch Factory, closes.

June 29, 1861
Genboku Itō amputates a gangrenous foot using chloroform. First recorded use of chloroform anesthesia in Japan.

January 1868 – June 1869

The Boshin War: a civil war in Japan triggered by the humili-ating aftermath of Commodore Perry's incursion.

1871

The last breast cancer operations on record at Shunrinken.

1882

Shunrinken hospital and medical school closes.

1899

The last known record of surgery with *Mafutsusan*.

1912

The Committee on Anesthesia of the American Medical Asso-ciation says that using chloroform as an anesthetic is no long-er justified, based on evidence for delayed poisoning.

May 1912

The first chloroform lawsuit in Japan.

1922

Dejima is designated a national historic site.

1923

Seishū Hanaoka and His Surgery by Shūzō Kure, the "bible" on Hanaoka, is published; it contains many errors. Shunrinken's main building is sold to a nearby village.

After World War II

Purple Cloud Ointment (*Shiunkō* in Japanese and *Tsiyúnkau* in Chinese), an antiseptic and anti-inflammatory skin remedy that promotes healthy blood circulation, is marketed in several countries. Developed in China in the seventeenth century, it was modified and improved by Hanaoka. It's still available.

1954

Hanaoka is inducted into the Hall of Fame of the International College of Surgeons in Chicago, IL.

Circa 1965

Chloroform is phased out in Japan.

1966

Anesthesiologist Akitomo Matsuki begins studying Hanaoka. He continues to discover new information.

1976

The U.S. Environmental Protection Agency labels chloroform a carcinogen.

1997

The Shunrinken building returns to Hanaoka's village, is rebuilt, and reopens as a museum. Dejima gets a museum too.

2000

October 13 is established in Japan as "Anesthesia Day" by the Japanese Society of Anesthesiologists (whose logo is an illustration of *Datura*), in accordance with Matsuki's proposal.

ACKNOWLEDGMENTS

Akitomo Matsuki entrusted me with this beautiful story, answered my questions promptly, and checked every detail for accuracy. During the two years we worked together, he said, "Facts can have numerous faces. A is A for one person, but B for another. Your writing will give me a chance to see a different face of Hanaoka. I am looking forward to reading it. . . . Your work will contribute to a better understanding of Seishū Hanaoka in western countries. . . . I was unable to find any trouble with your final version. It is perfect. . . . I think your success must come from both the eloquence of the sentences and the unfolding development of the story. It is due to your great skill in writing. I know your skill adequately because you have revised many English abstracts for me."

I discovered Nan Rae's art in a unique card shop – the kind people visit from miles around – in my hometown. Thinking one of her gorgeous paintings would look spectacular on the cover, I contacted her (it doesn't hurt to try). She was instantly enthusiastic about the project.

The Dutch Factory and the *Mafutsusan* plants were illustrated by my daughter Michelle's future mother-in-law, artist Gail Brill. Lucky for me, our children met in time for her exquisite drawings to be included.

I am inspired by my extraordinary daughters, Michelle and Eliza Kuchuk, to never give up on the creative life – because of their enthusiasm for anything I create, and because of the thoughtful creativity in their own lives.

Michelle also helped by reading a draft at the midway point. Her brilliant suggestions, which ran the gamut from tiny details to the big picture, improved the book tremendously.

Their dad, Fikri Kuchuk, a scientist who has published extensively, offered advice on citations and regaled me with stories of other scientific discoveries and inventions.

Bob Brodeur – printer, editor, and graphic designer – read an early draft and told me which parts were confusing or inconsistent. His insightful comments, along with the printing and tech stuff he did, were incredibly helpful.

The *very* long ether book title was translated from German to English by world traveler David Creighton.

My cats, Figment and Jinx, more or less followed my request not to race across or sleep on the keyboard while I worked.

Mary and John Bunker, my parents, never lost their curiosity. When a topic captured their interest (a common occurrence), there'd be a new surge of reading, writing, lectures, books on tape, and so on. By their example, I learned to be curious.

Thank you, all . . .

AUTHOR – COLLABORATOR – ARTISTS

Emily Bunker has a bachelor's degree in anthropology from Stanford University. She is a writer, editor, book designer, and enthusiastic puzzler. Her other recent book, *Pencil Lady*, is about her time as a high school math and physics tutor.

Akitomo Matsuki, Emeritus Professor of Anesthesiology at the Hirosaki University Graduate School of Medicine in Hirosaki, Japan, continues the search for pieces of Hanaoka's story. This is just one of his ongoing medical history projects.

The Matsuki Prize was created in 2009 to promote the study of the history of anesthesia in Japan, and to encourage members of the Japanese Society of Anesthesiologists, particularly young members, to study the subject.

"Romance of the Moon" (cover art) by **Nan Rae**

Internationally exhibited artist Nan Rae writes, lectures and teaches on Brush painting and Sumi-e.
nanraefineart.com nanraestudio.com

The significance of bamboo in Japanese culture . . .
It has a quality worth aspiring to: it bends but doesn't break.

My wife and I are greatly impressed with the cover. I deeply and sincerely think it symbolizes Hanaoka's mind.

– A. Matsuki

Mafutsusan plants and the Dutch Factory by **Gail Brill**

Gail lives in the Adirondack Mountains in New York State with her husband Jason, dog Jones and kitty Max. Gail has been a professional calligrapher and illustrator for 30 years and she counts her blessings daily. www.gailbrilldesign.com

Shunrinken student **Ryōkei Amenomori** originated the two illustrations of patients in the midst of breast cancer surgery. The versions here are replicas by his student **Sazen Inoue**.

The portrait of Seishū Hanaoka is by artist **Sogo Tanba**.

SOURCES

Almost all of the information in *And She Felt No Pain* originated with Dr. Akitomo Matsuki, either via our email exchange, from his article with Adolph H. Giesecke, "Hanaoka: The Great Master of Medicine, and His Book on Rare Diseases," *American Society of Anesthesiologists Newsletter* September 2008 <http://www.woodlibrarymuseum.org/news/newsletter/NL_2008.PDF#page=30> or from his books *Seishu Hanaoka and His Medicine: A Japanese Pioneer of Anesthesia and Surgery*; *A Short History of Anesthesia in Japan*; and *The Origin and Evolution of Anesthesia in Japan* (Hirosaki University Press, 2011, 2012, and 2017, respectively).

Additional Source Material

Quotations | *A distinguished American* . . . : Frank Preston Stearns, *Cambridge Sketches* (Kessinger Publishing, LLC, 2004; originally published in 1905) <http://www.authorama.com/cambridge-sketches-18.html> Accessed August 24, 2016.

Dedication | **British government . . ."what" or "how"**: Emily Gosden, "Nonsense! Backlash over new school rules on exclamation marks," *The Telegraph* March 6, 2016 <http://www.telegraph.co.uk/education/12185164/Nonsense-Backlash-over-new-school-rules-on-exclamation-marks.html> Accessed June 24, 2017.

1. Pain Free

3 | **Portrait of Seishū Hanaoka:** Shūzō Kure, *Seishū Hanaoka and His Surgery* (Tohōdō Shoten, 1923). Permission not required.

2. From Boyhood

4 | **In stark contrast . . . that gift:** John P. Bunker, personal communication.

3. Old-Style + Dutch-Style = Hanaoka-Style

9 | **"two systems of medicine . . .":** Subhuti Dharmananda, "Kampo Medicine: The Practice of Chinese Herbal Medicine in Japan," *Institute for Traditional Medicine* <http://www.itmonline.org/arts/kampo.htm> Accessed October 19, 2016.

11 | **blind Chinese priest . . . twelve years; excellent sense of smell . . . established; Over time . . . unproven theories:** Ibid.

12 | **Kulmus:** "Kulmus," *Historical Anatomies on the Web* <http://www.nlm.nih.gov/exhibition/historicalanatomies/kulmus_bio.html> Accessed November 12, 2016.

12 | **rooted in Confucianism:** N. S. Chu, "Legendary Hwa Tuo's surgery under general anesthesia in the second century China" (Acta Neurol Taiwan, December 2004), 211-6. Accessed November 12, 2016, from <http://www.ncbi.nlm.nih.gov/m/pubmed/15666698/>

13 | **"exit island":** "Dejima, Nagasaki," *Japan Visitor* <http://www.japanvisitor.com/japan-city-guides/dejima-nagasaki> Accessed August 8, 2017.

13 | **Dutch trading post . . . Compagnie:** Marc Jason Gilbert, "Paper Trails: Dejima Island: A Stepping Stone between Civilizations," *World History Connected* October 2006: par 3 <http://worldhistoryconnected.press.illinois.edu/3.3/gilbert.html> Accessed October 19, 2016.

13 | **bankrupt in 1796:** Ann Jannetta, *The Vaccinators: Smallpox, Medical Knowledge, and the 'Opening' of Japan* (Stanford University Press, 2007), 55.

13 | **Dutch flag:** "Dutch-Japanese Relations," *The Netherlands and You* <http://www.netherlandsandyou.nl/your-country-and-the-netherlands/japan/and-the-netherlands/dutch-japanese-relations> Accessed February 12, 2018.

13 | **twenty-four starving . . . James Clavell:** Gilbert, par 2.

14 | **The Portuguese . . . firearms:** Dieter Wanczura, "The Dutch in Nagasaki," *Artelino* March 2003 <http://www.artelino.com/articles/dutch_nagasaki.asp> Accessed October 19, 2016.

14 | **But when their interest . . . national security:** Kenneth Henshall, *A History of Japan: From Stone Age to Superpower* (Palgrave Macmillan, 2012), 59-61.

14 | **From 1792 to 1849 . . . castaways; Treaty of Kanagawa:** Ibid., 68-70.

14 | **Netherlands . . . ignored:** "Dutch-Japanese Relations," *The Netherlands and You.*

14-15 | **From the start . . . watchful eye:** Gilbert, pars 2-3.

15 | **According . . ."Like this!":** "Dejima, Nagasaki," *Japan Visitor.*

15 | **Thus began . . . Chinese silk:** "Dutch-Japanese Relations," *The Netherlands and You.*

15 | **Coffee:** Rochelle and Viet Hoang, "Coffee in Japan: 120 years of Mornings," *Tofugu* April 29, 2014 <http://www.tofugu.com/japan/japanese-coffee/> Accessed August 8, 2017.

15 | **Chocolate:** Rachel B, "Ch-Ch-Ch-Chocolate: Japan's Sudden Sweet," *Tofugu* September 4, 2013 <http://www.tofugu.com/japan/japanese-chocolate/> Accessed August 8, 2017.

15 | **Beer, badminton, and billiards:** "Dejima, Nagasaki," *Japan Visitor.*

15 | **Camera:** "A Short History of Photography in Japan," *KCP International: Japanese Language School* May 16, 2016 <http://www.kcpinternational.com/2016/05/a-short-history-of-photography-in-japan/> Accessed August 8, 2017.

15 | **their own trading:** "Dutch-Japanese Relations," *The Netherlands and You*.

15-16 | **periodic visit . . . offer gifts; bring news . . . primary function:** Gilbert, pars 3-4.

16 | **telescopes . . . kimonos:** "Dutch-Japanese Relations," *The Netherlands and You*.

16 | **Japanese artists . . . big noses:** Gilbert, par 12.

17 | **Caspar Schamberger:** "Caspar Schamberger's Life (1623-1706)," *History of Cultural Contacts Europe – East Asia* <http://wolfgangmichel.web.fc2.com/serv/cs/cs-chronology-engl.html> Accessed February 12, 2018.

17 | **Engelbert Kaempfer:** Gilbert, pars 21-22.

17 | **doctors had more freedom:** Jannetta, 88.

17 | **Siebold Incident:** Ibid., 94. Ann Jannetta says, "For a summary account of the Siebold Incident, see Conrad Totman, *Early Modern Japan* (University of California Press, 1993), 509-511."

18 | **ability to read . . . Latin alphabet:** Ibid., 126-27.

18 | **worth the trouble . . . improve lives:** Ibid., 3.

4. Fish Hooks or Finger Traps

19-20 | **Chinese finger trap:** Oliver Burkeman, *The Antidote: Happiness for People Who Can't Stand Positive Thinking* (Faber and Faber, Inc., 2012), 21-22.

6. Six Potent Plants

31 | **Alkaloids . . . anesthetic properties:** The Editors of Encyclopædia Britannica, "Alkaloid: Chemical Compound," *Britannica* <http://www.britannica.com/science/alkaloid> Accessed May 23, 2017.

32, 34, 36, 38 | **The plants of *Mafutsusan*:** By permission of Plants For A Future <http://pfaf.org> Accessed January 12, 2017. *The main aims of the charity are researching and providing information on ecologically sustainable horticulture, as an integral part of designs involving high species diversity and permaculture principles.*

7. Testing, Testing

41 | **Self-experimentation . . . chloroform:** John P. Bunker, personal communication.

9. Then the People Come

62-63 | **Illustrations of surgery patients:** By permission of the Kannon Museum, Nagahama, Japan.

12. Going Dutch

82 | Boshin War . . . forced opening: Henshall, 70, 76, 236.

82 | trichloromethane . . . compound; still in use . . . from *Datura*: "Chloroform," *National Center for Biotechnology Information.* Pubchem Compound Database; CID=6212 <http://pubchem.ncbi.nlm.nih.gov/compound/6212> Accessed March 26, 2017.

82-83 | forty times sweeter . . . sedatives; synthesized . . . March 1847: "Chloroform," *Medical Discoveries* <http://www.discoveriesinmedicine.com/Bar-Cod/Chloroform.html> Accessed March 31, 2017.

83 | Eight months . . . footnote of history: Keith Sykes, with John Bunker, Contributing Editor, *Anaesthesia and the Practice of Medicine: Historical Perspectives* (Royal Society of Medicine Press Ltd, 2007), 16-17, 19.

83-84 | sprinkled . . . opted for the pain: "Ether and Chloroform," *History* <http://www.history.com/topics/ether-and-chloroform> Accessed March 31, 2017.

84 | A 15-year-old girl . . . however: Sykes and Bunker, 19.

84 | Queen Victoria . . . giving birth: Ibid., 250.

84-85 | Ether and nitrous oxide . . . Crawford W. Long; October 16 . . . of each other: Ibid., 9-12.

85 | **Horace Wells and John M. Riggs:** Richard J. Wolfe, "Who Was the Discoverer of Surgical Anesthesia? A Brief for Horace Wells," *I Awaken to Glory: Essays Celebrating Horace Wells and the Sesquicentennial of the Discovery of Anesthesia, December 11, 1844 – December 11, 1994*, edited by Richard J. Wolfe and Leonard F. Menczer (The Francis A. Countway Library of Medicine, Boston, in Association with The Historical Museum of Medicine and Dentistry, Hartford, 1994), 2.

85 | **Possibly earlier than Dec. 11:** Horace Wells, *History of the Discovery of the Application of Nitrous Oxide Gas, Ether, and other Vapors, to Surgical Operations* (Reprint; originally published by J. Gaylord Wells in Hartford, 1847), 15, 18, 33, 35.

85 | **Wells *put himself under*:** David A. Chernin, "Genius, the Result of Original Mental Superiority: John M. Riggs and Horace Wells," Wolfe and Menczer, 262.

85 | **but only Wells . . . money from it:** J. A. W. Wildsmith, "Recognition from Britain: The Horace Wells Testimonial Fund, 1871-1873," Ibid., 302.

85 | **"I was desirous . . .":** Wells, 25.

86 | **caught the ear of the establishment:** Truman Smith, *An Examination of the Question of Anaesthesia* (1853), 63 <https://archive.org/details/examinationofque00smit> Accessed October 22, 2019.

88 | **administered . . . failed attempts:** Jannetta, 132-33.

90 | **Oliver Wendell Holmes Sr.:** "Ether and Chloroform," *History*.

91 | **he broke from . . . Paris:** Jannetta, 175.

91 | **Ine Kusumoto:** "Kusumoto Ine: The First Female Doctor of Western Medicine in Japan," *Up Closed* <http://upclosed.com/people/kusumoto-ine> Accessed February 12, 2018.

94 | **American surgeons . . . effective anesthetics:** "Ether and Chloroform," *History*.

94 | **depress most organs; carcinogen:** "Chloroform," *Medical Discoveries*.

94 | **cardiac death and liver failure:** Sykes and Bunker, 221.

94 | **Committee on Anesthesia . . . poisoning:** Ibid., 226.

13. What Happens Next

95 | **consulate . . . underway:** "Dejima Comes Back to Life," <http://www.city.nagasaki.lg.jp/dejima/en/history/conten ts/frame_006_001.html> Accessed April 17, 2017.

Timeline

107 | **Purple Cloud Ointment . . . improved by Hanaoka:** Dharmananda.

Made in the USA
Lexington, KY
14 November 2019